Ayurveda & Modern Dermatology

(Diagnosis and Treatment of Skin Disorders)

Dr. Mukesh Aggarwal

Preface

In the realm of dermatology, bridging the timeless wisdom of Ayurveda with the advancements of modern medicine marks a significant stride towards comprehensive skin care. This book, "Ayurvedic & Modern Dermatology: Diagnosis and Treatment of Skin Disorders," is born out of a passionate endeavor to fuse these two streams of knowledge, offering a holistic approach to understanding and addressing skin ailments.

As an Ayurveda Physician, I deeply rooted in both Ayurveda and modern medicine, I have witnessed the profound insights each tradition brings to the diagnosis and treatment of skin disorders. Ayurveda, with its intricate understanding of doshas and holistic healing principles, complements the precision and innovation of modern dermatology.

In this book, we embark on a journey through the intricacies of skin health, exploring the fundamental concepts of Ayurveda alongside contemporary medical perspectives. From the classification and diagnosis of skin disorders to the modalities used in treatment, each chapter is meticulously crafted to provide a comprehensive understanding of the subject matter.

Furthermore, the inclusion of specific skin disorders, along with their Ayurvedic and modern treatment modalities, serves as a practical guide for both practitioners and individuals seeking holistic skin care solutions. Additionally, the chapter on holistic skin care practices emphasizes the importance of daily routines, seasonal adjustments, and mind-body practices in maintaining optimal skin health.

Moreover, the vision for the future outlined in the final chapters underscores the potential for further integration and collaboration between Ayurvedic and modern dermatology, paving the way for innovative approaches to skin care.

It is my sincere hope that this book serves as a valuable resource for Ayurvedic practitioners, and individuals alike, fostering a deeper appreciation for the synergies between ancient wisdom and contemporary science in the pursuit of radiant skin health.

Dr. Mukesh Aggarwal

Acknowledgments

I would like to express my deepest gratitude to all those who have contributed to the realization of this book, "Ayurvedic & Modern Dermatology: Diagnosis and Treatment of Skin Disorders."

First and foremost, I am indebted to my teachers and mentors whose guidance and wisdom have shaped my understanding of dermatology, both from the perspectives of Ayurveda and modern medicine. Their invaluable insights have enriched this book and have been instrumental in its creation.

I extend heartfelt thanks to the patients who have entrusted me with their care and shared their experiences, serving as a source of inspiration and learning. Your trust and cooperation have been essential in deepening my understanding of skin disorders and refining the approaches discussed in this book.

I am grateful to my colleagues and peers for their support, encouragement, and collaborative spirit throughout this journey. Their diverse perspectives and expertise have contributed significantly to the breadth and depth of the content presented in this book.

Special appreciation goes to my family for their unwavering support, understanding, and patience during the countless hours devoted to research, writing, and editing. Your love and encouragement have been my greatest motivation.

Last but not least, I extend my sincere thanks to the readers of this book. It is my hope that the knowledge shared within these pages will empower you to understand and address skin disorders effectively, thereby promoting health and well-being.

Dr Mukesh Aggarwal

Contents

Cheilitis (ओष्ठपाक)
Chicken Pox (लघुमसुरिका)
Corn (अट्टन)
Dandruff (दारुणक)
Dermatitis (क्षुद्र कुष्ठ)
Eczema (विचर्चिका)
Erysipelas (विसर्प)
Freckles (तिल)
Folliculitis (रोमकूपशोथ)
Greying of Hair (पालित्य)
Hair Fall (खालित्य)
Heel Fissure (विपादक)
Herpes (हर्पिस)
Hyperhidrosis (श्वेद आधिक्य)
Impetigo (पानीवात)
Insect Bite (कीड़ा काटना)
Itchyosis (इचियोसिस)
Keloid (किलोइड)
Leprosy (कुष्ठ)
Leukoplakia (मुंह में सफेद दाग)
Lichen Planus (लाइकेन प्लानस)
Lipoma (चर्बी की गांठ)
Lupus (ल्युपस)
Melasma (छाइयाँ)
Moles (तिलकालक)
Morphea (त्वक काठिन्य)
Onychomycosis (नखकवकता)
Paronychia (नखपाक)
Pediculosis (जुएं)
Pellegra (पेलग्रा)
Pemphigus (पेम्फीगस)
Prickly Heat (घमोरियां)
Pruritus (कंडु)
Psoriasis (शिघ्म कुष्ठ)

Pityriasis (पीटीरिअसिस)
Rosacea (रोजेशिया)
Scabies (पामा)
Stomatitis (मुखपाक)
Tinea (फफूंदी)
Urticaria (शीतपित्त)
Vitiligo (श्वेतकुष्ठ)
Warts (चर्मकील)
Whitlow (कुनख चिप्प)

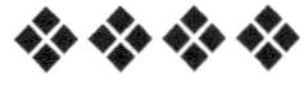

Chapter 1

UNDERSTANDING SKIN

Skin According to Ayurveda Science

According to Ayurveda, there are seven types of skin, known as "prakriti," each with its own unique characteristics:

Vata Skin: Vata skin tends to be dry, thin, delicate, and cool to the touch. It is prone to fine lines, wrinkles, and premature aging due to lack of moisture and oil. People with Vata skin may experience flakiness, roughness, and sensitivity.

Pitta Skin: Pitta skin is fair, sensitive, and prone to inflammation and redness. It can be warm to the touch and may develop conditions like acne, rosacea, and eczema when out of balance. Pitta skin tends to have medium thickness and is prone to sunburn.

Kapha Skin: Kapha skin is typically oily, thick, and smooth. It has a natural glow and is more resilient to wrinkles and aging. However, Kapha skin is prone to clogged pores, blackheads, and acne due to excess oil production.

Vata-Pitta Skin: Vata-Pitta skin combines the characteristics of both Vata and Pitta skin types. It tends to be dry, sensitive, and prone to inflammation. Individuals with this skin type may experience a combination of dryness, redness, and irritation.

Vata-Kapha Skin: Vata-Kapha skin combines the qualities of Vata and Kapha skin types. It is typically dry and sensitive with occasional oiliness. This skin type may experience fluctuating conditions, such as dryness in some areas and oiliness in others.

Pitta-Kapha Skin: Pitta-Kapha skin combines the characteristics of Pitta and Kapha skin types. It is often oily, sensitive, and prone to inflammation and congestion. Individuals with this skin type may experience a combination of oiliness, redness, and occasional breakouts.

Tridoshic Skin: Tridoshic skin is a balance of all three doshas – Vata, Pitta, and Kapha. It is typically radiant, clear, and well-hydrated. People with Tridoshic skin often have minimal skin issues and a healthy complexion.

Understanding your skin type according to Ayurveda can help tailor skincare routines and dietary choices to maintain balance and promote overall well-being.

Layers of Skin According to Ayurveda

In Ayurveda, the skin is described as having seven layers.

Avabhasini: This is the outermost layer of the skin, representing the epidermis. It acts as a protective barrier against external factors such as pollution, pathogens, and UV radiation.

Lohita: Lohita corresponds to the blood vessels and capillaries in the skin. It is responsible for supplying nutrients and oxygen to the skin cells, promoting overall health and vitality.

Shweta: Shweta refers to the layer of the skin that contains the sweat glands and hair follicles. It regulates body temperature through perspiration and helps to eliminate toxins from the body.

Tamra: Tamra represents the layer of the skin that contains melanin, giving the skin its color. It also plays a role in protecting the skin from harmful UV radiation and regulating pigmentation.

Vedini: Vedini corresponds to the nerve endings in the skin. It is responsible for transmitting sensory information such as touch, temperature, and pain perception.

Rohini: Rohini is the layer of the skin that contains the lymphatic vessels. It helps to remove waste products and toxins from the skin, supporting detoxification and immune function.

Mamsadhara: It represents the deepest layer of the skin, containing muscles and connective tissue. It provides structural support and stability to the skin, helping to maintain its firmness and elasticity.
Understanding the different layers of the skin according to Ayurveda can provide insight into its functions and help guide skincare practices to promote overall health and well-being.

Skin According to Modern Medicine

Introduction: The skin, the body's largest organ, serves as a protective barrier between the internal organs and the external environment. Its complex structure enables it to fulfill various functions crucial for maintaining homeostasis and protecting against external threats.

Layers of The Skin: The skin comprises three primary layers: the epidermis, dermis, and hypodermis (subcutaneous tissue). Each layer plays a distinct role in the overall function of the skin.

Epidermis: The outermost layer of the skin.

Composed mainly of keratinocytes, which produce the protein keratin, providing strength and waterproofing.

Contains melanocytes, responsible for producing melanin, which gives skin its color and protects against UV radiation.

Also includes Langerhans cells, part of the immune system, and Merkel cells, which are involved in sensation.

Dermis: Lies beneath the epidermis and is significantly thicker.

Comprises connective tissue rich in collagen and elastin fibers, providing strength, elasticity, and support.

Contains blood vessels, lymphatic vessels, nerve endings, hair follicles, and sweat glands.

Responsible for regulating temperature, sensation, and supplying nutrients to the skin.

Hypodermis: Also known as the subcutaneous tissue.
Consists of adipose (fat) tissue and connective tissue.
Acts as an energy reservoir, insulation, and shock absorber.

Connects the skin to underlying muscles and bones.

Structural Components: Several structural components contribute to the integrity and function of the skin.

Hair Follicles: Invaginations of the epidermis into the dermis.

Produce hair and associated structures such as sebaceous glands (secrete sebum) and arrector pili muscles (responsible for hair erection).

Sweat Glands:

Eccrine Glands: Distributed throughout the body and produce sweat for thermoregulation.

Apocrine Glands: Found in areas such as the axillae and groin, producing a thicker secretion that is odorless but can become odorous when metabolized by skin bacteria.

Blood Vessels: Provide nutrients and oxygen to the skin.
Regulate body temperature through vasodilation and vasoconstriction.

Importance of Skin Health

Skin, the largest organ of the human body, plays a pivotal role not only in protecting our internal organs but also in reflecting our overall health. From shielding us against external threats to regulating body temperature, skin health is paramount for maintaining a robust immune system and overall well-being.

Following Are the Functions of Skin

Protection: Skin acts as a barrier, safeguarding our body against harmful pathogens, UV radiation, and environmental toxins. Intact skin prevents infections and reduces the risk of diseases.

Thermoregulation: Through processes like sweating and vasodilation, skin helps regulate body temperature, ensuring optimal physiological functioning. Maintaining a balanced temperature is vital for metabolic processes and overall comfort.

Sensation: Skin is equipped with sensory receptors that allow us to perceive touch, pressure, temperature, and pain. These sensations are crucial for detecting potential dangers and maintaining spatial awareness.

Vitamin D Synthesis: Exposure to sunlight enables the synthesis of vitamin D in the skin. This essential vitamin plays a key role in bone health, immune function, and mood regulation.

Hydration and Barrier Function: Proper hydration is essential for maintaining skin elasticity and suppleness. Additionally, the skin's lipid barrier prevents excessive water loss and protects against irritants and allergens.

Psychological Well-Being: The appearance of our skin can significantly impact our self-esteem and mental health. Healthy skin contributes to a positive body image and enhances confidence and social interactions.

Early Detection of Health Issues: Changes in the skin's appearance or texture can be indicative of underlying health conditions such as allergies, hormonal imbalances, or systemic diseases. Regular skin examinations can aid in the early detection and management of these issues.

Wound Healing: Skin plays a crucial role in the wound healing process. It forms a protective barrier over injuries, facilitates tissue repair, and reduces the risk of infection. Maintaining skin health is essential for efficient wound healing and scar prevention.

Conclusion: the importance of skin health cannot be overstated. Beyond its role as a physical barrier, skin influences various aspects of our well-being, from immune function to psychological state. By prioritizing skin care practices and seeking prompt medical attention for any abnormalities, individuals can maintain optimal skin health and enjoy a higher quality of life.

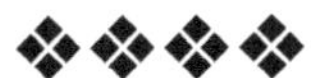

Chapter 2

CLASSIFICATION OF SKIN DISORDERS

Classification of Skin Disorders According to Ayurveda

Ayurveda, an ancient system of medicine originating from the Indian subcontinent, offers a comprehensive understanding of skin disorders based on the principles of Tridosha theory, Panchamahabhutas (five elements), and Saptadhatu (seven tissues). Skin disorders in Ayurveda are classified primarily based on the imbalance of the three doshas: Vata, Pitta, and Kapha.

Vata-Related Skin Disorders:

Vata governs the elements of air and ether, responsible for mobility and dryness. Skin disorders associated with Vata imbalance often manifest as dryness, roughness, and cracking.

EXAMPLES INCLUDE:

Vicharchika (Eczema): Characterized by dry, itchy patches on the skin, often aggravated by stress and improper diet.

Pittajashtim (Psoriasis): Presents as thick, scaly patches with inflammation, aggravated by stress and spicy foods.

Pitta-Related Skin Disorders:

Pitta, representing fire and water elements, governs metabolism and digestion. Pitta imbalance leads to excessive heat and inflammation in the body, reflecting in the skin.

EXAMPLES INCLUDE:

Pama (acne): Resulting from excess oil production and inflammation, aggravated by spicy and oily foods, stress, and hormonal fluctuations.

Dadru (fungal infections): Presents as circular patches with itching and redness, exacerbated by poor hygiene and excessive sweating.

KAPHA-RELATED SKIN DISORDERS:

Kapha, associated with earth and water elements, governs structure and lubrication in the body. Kapha imbalance leads to excess oiliness and heaviness in the skin.

EXAMPLES INCLUDE:

Kandu (Urticaria): Characterized by raised, itchy welts on the skin, triggered by allergens and cold weather.

Kshudra Kushtha (Minor Skin Disorders): Encompasses various minor skin conditions like warts, cysts, and skin tags, often aggravated by poor diet and lifestyle.

Conclusion: In Ayurveda, the classification of skin disorders is intricately linked to the balance of the doshas and their influence on skin health. By addressing the underlying imbalances through holistic approaches, Ayurveda offers effective solutions for treating various skin conditions and promoting overall well-being.

Classification of Skin Disorders According to Modern Medicine

Modern medicine classifies skin disorders based on various factors such as their etiology, symptoms, and histopathological characteristics. Here's a detailed classification of skin disorders according to modern medicine:

Infectious Skin Disorders:

Bacterial Infections: Including impetigo, cellulitis, and folliculitis.

Viral Infections: Such as herpes simplex, herpes zoster (shingles), and warts.

Fungal Infections: Including ringworm (tinea corporis), athlete's foot (tinea pedis), and candidiasis.

Parasitic Infections: Such as scabies and lice infestations.

Inflammatory Skin Disorders:

Eczematous Disorders: Such as atopic dermatitis, contact dermatitis, and seborrheic dermatitis.

Psoriasis: Characterized by red, scaly patches on the skin, often with associated joint inflammation (psoriatic arthritis).

LUPUS Erythematosus: Including discoid lupus erythematosus and systemic lupus erythematosus (SLE).

Acne Vulgaris: A common disorder characterized by comedones, papules, pustules, and nodules.

Allergic Skin Disorders:

Urticaria (Hives): Characterized by raised, itchy welts on the skin, often triggered by allergens.

Angioedema: Involving deeper swelling in the skin, often affecting the face, lips, and eyelids.

Allergic Contact Dermatitis: Resulting from exposure to allergens such as metals, fragrances, and plants.

Neoplastic Skin Disorders:

Basal Cell Carcinoma: The most common type of skin cancer, usually presenting as a pearly or waxy bump.

Squamous Cell Carcinoma: Arising from squamous cells in the epidermis, often appearing as a red, scaly patch or a firm, red nodule.

Melanoma: A potentially deadly form of skin cancer originating from melanocytes, often presenting as an irregularly shaped mole with asymmetrical borders and variegated color.

Pigmentary Disorders:

Vitiligo: Characterized by depigmented patches on the skin due to the destruction of melanocytes.

Hyperpigmentation: Including conditions like melasma, post-inflammatory hyperpigmentation, and lentigines (age spots).

Autoimmune Skin Disorders:

Pemphigus: Characterized by blistering of the skin and mucous membranes due to autoantibodies targeting desmosomes.

Bullous Pemphigoid: Involving tense blisters and urticarial plaques, often associated with autoantibodies against hemidesmosomes.

Genodermatoses:

Ichthyosis: Characterized by dry, scaly skin due to abnormal keratinization.

Epidermolysis Bullosa: Inherited disorders characterized by blistering of the skin and mucous membranes in response to minor trauma.

Xeroderma Pigmentosum: A rare genetic disorder predisposing individuals to skin cancer due to defective DNA repair mechanisms.

Vascular Skin Disorders:

Varicose Veins: Enlarged, twisted veins usually occurring in the legs, causing discomfort and cosmetic concerns.

Hemangiomas: Benign tumors composed of blood vessels, often present at birth and regressing with age.

Telangiectasias: Small, dilated blood vessels near the surface of the skin, commonly seen in conditions like rosacea and spider veins.

Conclusion: Modern medicine provides a comprehensive classification of skin disorders based on various factors, including infectious agents, inflammatory processes, neoplastic changes, autoimmune reactions, genetic predispositions, and vascular abnormalities. Understanding these classifications aids in accurate diagnosis and management of skin conditions, promoting optimal patient care and outcomes.

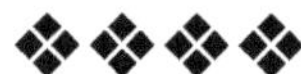

DIAGNOSIS OF SKIN DISORDERS

Diagnosis of Skin Disorders According to Ayurveda Science

Understanding Doshas: Vata, Pitta, And Kapha in Relations of Skin Disorders

Introduction: Ayurveda, revolves around the concept of doshas – Vata, Pitta, and Kapha. These doshas are believed to govern various physiological and psychological functions of the body, including skin health. Understanding their influence on skin disorders provides valuable insights into holistic approaches for treatment and prevention.

Vata Dosha and Skin Disorders: Vata, composed of air and ether elements, governs movement and communication in the body. When imbalanced, it can manifest in dryness, roughness, and sensitivity, leading to skin disorders such as eczema, psoriasis, and dry skin. Vata-related skin issues often worsen during dry and windy weather conditions. Balancing Vata through nourishing oils, warm and grounding foods, and gentle lifestyle practices can help alleviate these conditions.

Pitta Dosha and Skin Disorders: Pitta, associated with fire and water elements, governs metabolism and transformation. Imbalanced Pitta can lead to inflammation, redness, and sensitivity in the skin, resulting in conditions like acne, rosacea, and rashes. Pitta-related skin issues often flare up with exposure to heat and spicy foods. Cooling and calming remedies, such as hydrating herbal teas, cooling herbs like aloe vera, and avoiding hot and spicy foods, can help pacify Pitta and promote skin healing.

Kapha Dosha and Skin Disorders: Kapha, comprising earth and water elements, governs structure and lubrication in the body. When aggravated, Kapha can lead to excess oiliness, congestion, and stagnation in the skin, contributing to conditions like oily skin, cystic acne, and comedones. Kapha-related skin issues tend to worsen during cold and damp weather conditions. Balancing Kapha through cleansing herbs, light and warm foods, and regular exercise can help prevent and manage these skin disorders.

Conclusion: Understanding the influence of Vata, Pitta, and Kapha doshas on skin disorders provides valuable insights for personalized and holistic approaches to treatment and prevention. By addressing imbalances in the doshas through lifestyle modifications, herbal remedies, and natural skincare practices, individuals can promote optimal skin health and overall well-being in alignment with the principles of Ayurveda.

Pulse Diagnosis and Tongue Examination in Skin Disorders

Ayurveda employs unique diagnostic methods such as pulse diagnosis (Nadi Pariksha) and tongue examination (Jivha Pariksha) to assess imbalances in the body, including those related to skin disorders. These traditional techniques offer valuable insights into an individual's constitution, dosha status, and underlying causes of skin ailments, enabling personalized treatment approaches for optimal healing.

Pulse Diagnosis (Nadi Pariksha) And Skin Disorders: Pulse diagnosis is a sophisticated technique in Ayurveda where the practitioner assesses the subtle qualities of the pulse to determine the balance or imbalance of the three doshas – Vata, Pitta, and Kapha. In the context of skin disorders, specific pulse characteristics may indicate imbalances associated with each dosha. For instance, a rapid and erratic pulse may suggest Vata imbalance, while a strong and bounding pulse could signify Pitta aggravation. Similarly, a slow and sluggish pulse may indicate Kapha dominance. By analyzing pulse patterns and assessing the rhythm, strength, and quality of the pulse, Ayurvedic practitioners can gain insights into the root causes of skin disorders and tailor treatment protocols accordingly.

Tongue Examination (Jivha Pariksha) And Skin Disorders: Tongue examination is another integral aspect of Ayurvedic diagnosis that provides valuable information about an individual's health status, including imbalances affecting the skin. In Jivha Pariksha, the practitioner observes the color, coating, moisture, and overall appearance of the tongue to assess dosha imbalances and associated health conditions. In the context of skin disorders, certain tongue characteristics may correlate with specific dosha imbalances. For example, a dry and cracked tongue coating may indicate Vata imbalance, while a yellowish or reddish tongue with a prominent coating could suggest Pitta aggravation. Additionally, a thick white coating on the tongue may signify Kapha dominance. By interpreting tongue signs in conjunction with other diagnostic methods, Ayurvedic practitioners can gain a comprehensive understanding of an individual's constitution and tailor treatment strategies to address skin imbalances effectively.

Integration of Diagnostic Methods: In Ayurveda, pulse diagnosis and tongue examination are often integrated with other diagnostic techniques, such as observation of physical characteristics (Darshanam), inquiry into lifestyle habits (Prashna), and assessment of bodily functions (Sparshanam), to form a comprehensive diagnostic approach. By considering multiple aspects of an individual's health and analyzing subtle indicators of dosha imbalances, practitioners can develop personalized treatment plans that target the underlying causes of skin disorders. Holistic interventions encompassing dietary modifications, lifestyle adjustments, herbal remedies, and therapeutic practices aim to restore balance and promote optimal skin health according to Ayurvedic principles.

Conclusion: Pulse diagnosis and tongue examination are invaluable diagnostic tools in Ayurveda for assessing imbalances related to skin disorders. By skillfully interpreting pulse patterns and tongue characteristics, practitioners can identify underlying dosha imbalances and tailor treatment protocols to address the root causes of skin ailments. Integrating these traditional diagnostic methods with holistic interventions facilitates personalized care and promotes long-term skin wellness in alignment with Ayurvedic Examination.

Identifying Triggers and Aggravating Factors of Skin Disorders

In Ayurveda, understanding the triggers and aggravating factors of skin disorders is crucial for effective management and prevention. By recognizing the environmental, dietary, lifestyle, and emotional influences that contribute to imbalances in the doshas — Vata, Pitta, and Kapha — practitioners can provide personalized interventions to restore harmony and promote skin health.

Environmental Factors: Environmental factors play a significant role in the development and exacerbation of skin disorders according to Ayurveda. Exposure to dry and windy weather conditions can aggravate Vata dosha, leading to dryness, roughness, and sensitivity in the skin. Similarly, excessive heat and sunlight can exacerbate Pitta dosha, causing inflammation, redness, and irritation. Cold and damp conditions, on the other hand, can worsen Kapha imbalances, resulting in excess oiliness and congestion in the skin. By identifying environmental triggers and recommending protective measures such as appropriate clothing, moisturizers, and sunscreens, Ayurvedic practitioners can help mitigate the impact of environmental factors on skin health.

Dietary Factors: Dietary factors play a significant role in Ayurveda in the development and management of skin disorders. Consuming foods that aggravate specific doshas can exacerbate skin imbalances and contribute to the onset of symptoms. For example, spicy, oily, and fried foods can exacerbate Pitta dosha, leading to inflammation and acne. Dry and light foods can aggravate Vata dosha, causing dryness and roughness in the skin. Heavy and dense foods, such as dairy products and sweets, can worsen Kapha imbalances, resulting in oiliness and congestion. By identifying dietary triggers and recommending a balanced diet tailored to individual dosha imbalances, Ayurvedic practitioners can support skin health from within.

Lifestyle Factors: Lifestyle factors, including stress, sleep patterns, and physical activity levels, play a significant role in Ayurveda in the development and management of skin disorders. Chronic stress and inadequate sleep can disturb the balance of the doshas, weaken the immune system, and exacerbate skin conditions. Sedentary lifestyles and lack of exercise can aggravate Kapha dosha, leading to stagnation and congestion in the skin. By promoting stress management techniques, healthy sleep hygiene, and regular exercise, Ayurvedic practitioners can help individuals maintain balance and resilience in the face of lifestyle-related triggers.

Emotional Factors: Emotional factors, such as anxiety, anger, and fear, can profoundly influence skin health according to Ayurveda. Emotional imbalances can disrupt the flow of prana (life force energy) in the body, leading to disturbances in the doshas and manifesting as skin disorders. Stressful life events, unresolved emotions, and negative thought patterns can exacerbate existing skin conditions or trigger flare-ups. By addressing underlying emotional imbalances through techniques such as meditation, mindfulness, and counseling, Ayurvedic practitioners can support holistic healing and promote emotional well-being, which is closely linked to skin health.

Conclusion: Identifying triggers and aggravating factors of skin disorders is essential in Ayurveda for effective management and prevention. By recognizing the influence of environmental, dietary, lifestyle, and emotional factors on dosha imbalances, practitioners can offer personalized interventions to restore balance and promote skin health. Holistic approaches encompassing protective measures, dietary modifications, lifestyle adjustments, and emotional well-being techniques aim to address the root causes of skin disorders and support long-term healing according to Ayurvedic principles.

Viruddha Ahara and Its Impact On Skin Disorders

Ayurveda emphasizes the intimate connection between diet and health. Viruddha Ahara, or incompatible food combinations, is a key concept in Ayurveda that highlights how improper dietary habits can lead to various health issues, including skin disorders. Understanding Viruddha Ahara and its implications for skin health is essential for maintaining overall well-being.

In Ayurveda, the skin is considered a reflection of one's internal health, and imbalances in the body can manifest as skin disorders. Viruddha Ahara disrupts the balance of doshas (bioenergies) in the body, leading to the accumulation of toxins (ama) and aggravation of skin conditions. Let's explore some common examples of Viruddha Ahara in relation to skin disorders:

Contradictory Food Combinations: Ayurveda advises against consuming foods with contradictory properties, such as combining hot and cold foods or mixing heavy and light foods. These incompatible combinations can disturb digestion and metabolism, leading to toxin accumulation in the body. Over time, this can manifest as various skin issues like acne, eczema, and rashes.

Improper Food Pairings: Certain food combinations, such as milk with sour fruits or fish with dairy, are considered incompatible in Ayurveda. Consuming these combinations can lead to digestive disturbances and aggravate skin disorders. For example, mixing milk with citrus fruits can create an acidic environment in the stomach, which may exacerbate conditions like psoriasis and dermatitis.

Overeating or Under-Eating: Irregular eating habits, such as overeating or under-eating, can disrupt the digestive process and lead to the accumulation of toxins in the body. This can result in skin issues like dullness, dryness, and acne. Ayurveda emphasizes the importance of moderation in eating to maintain proper digestion and skin health.

Processed and Junk Foods: Ayurveda warns against the consumption of processed and junk foods, which are often high in unhealthy fats, sugars, and artificial additives. These foods can weaken digestion, increase toxin accumulation, and contribute to skin problems like acne, inflammation, and premature aging.

Inadequate Hydration: Insufficient water intake can impair digestion and detoxification processes in the body, leading to toxin accumulation and skin disorders. Proper hydration is essential for maintaining skin elasticity, moisture, and overall health. Ayurveda recommends drinking warm water throughout the day to support digestion and cleanse toxins from the body.

Unfavorable Eating Practices: Eating while stressed, distracted, or in a hurry can hinder proper digestion and assimilation of nutrients, leading to toxin buildup and skin issues. Ayurveda emphasizes the importance of mindful eating in a calm and peaceful environment to optimize digestion and promote skin health.

Types of Viruddha Ahara

Samanak Viruddha: This type of incompatibility arises when two or more substances with similar properties or qualities are combined. For example, mixing hot and hot substances, such as honey and ghee, can lead to an aggravation of Pitta dosha, causing digestive issues or skin problems.

Viparita Viruddha: Viparita Viruddha occurs when opposite substances are combined. This includes mixing hot and cold substances or incompatible tastes, such as consuming milk with fish. Such combinations can impair digestion, create toxins (ama), and disturb the dosha balance in the body.

Kala Viruddha: Kala Viruddha refers to the improper timing of consuming certain substances. For instance, consuming heavy or difficult-to-digest foods during the wrong time of day, such as having a heavy meal late at night, can lead to digestive discomfort and disrupt the body's natural rhythm.

Desha Viruddha: Desha Viruddha pertains to consuming substances inappropriate for the environment or geographical location. For example, consuming tropical fruits in a cold climate can weaken digestion and aggravate Vata dosha, leading to gas, bloating, and other Vata-related issues.

Agni Viruddha: Agni Viruddha occurs when substances incompatible with an individual's digestive fire (agni) are consumed. This can include consuming foods that are too heavy, too light, or difficult to digest for one's constitution. For instance, someone with a weak digestive fire should avoid heavy, oily foods that can overwhelm their digestion.

Matra Viruddha: Matra Viruddha refers to the improper dosage or quantity of substances consumed. Consuming too much or too little of a particular substance can disrupt the body's balance and lead to health issues. For example, excessive intake of spices or salt can aggravate Pitta dosha and cause acidity or inflammation.

Let's Explore Some Viruddha Ahara and Their Implications for Skin Health.

Milk and Salt: Consuming milk with salt can disturb the balance of doshas (bioenergies) in the body, leading to skin issues like acne and eczema.

Milk and Sour Fruits: Combining milk with sour fruits like citrus fruits can cause digestive problems and aggravate skin disorders such as psoriasis and dermatitis.

Honey and Ghee in Equal Quantities: Although individually beneficial, combining honey and ghee in equal proportions can produce toxins in the body, affecting skin health negatively.

Radish and Milk: Consuming radish with milk can lead to digestive issues and may exacerbate skin conditions like rashes and itching.

Fish and Milk: The combination of fish and milk is considered incompatible in Ayurveda and can lead to toxin formation in the body, manifesting as skin eruptions and allergies.

Yogurt and Fruit: Mixing yogurt with fruits can impair digestion and contribute to skin problems such as acne and inflammation.

Sesame Oil and Honey: Combining sesame oil with honey can lead to toxin formation in the body, affecting skin health adversely.

Banana with Buttermilk: Consuming banana with buttermilk may lead to indigestion and worsen skin conditions like eczema and psoriasis.

Hot and Cold Foods Together: Eating hot and cold foods together can disturb the digestive fire (agni), leading to toxin accumulation and skin disorders such as hives and itching.

Fish and Yogurt: Combining fish with yogurt can impair digestion and contribute to skin issues like acne and rosacea.

Cheese and Fruit: Consuming cheese with fruits can lead to fermentation in the gut, causing toxin formation and skin problems like acne and eczema.

Radish and Honey: Mixing radish with honey can disrupt digestion and contribute to skin ailments such as rashes and itching.

Lemon with Milk: Consuming lemon with milk can curdle the milk and disturb digestion, potentially leading to skin issues like acne and hives.

Nightshade Vegetables and Dairy: Nightshade vegetables like tomatoes and dairy products may not combine well and can exacerbate skin conditions such as eczema and psoriasis.

Fruits with Starches: Consuming fruits with starches like rice or bread can lead to fermentation in the gut, causing toxin formation and skin problems like acne and dermatitis.

Meat with Starches: Combining meat with starches can lead to impaired digestion and toxin accumulation, affecting skin health negatively.

Sour Fruits with Milk: Mixing sour fruits with milk can disrupt digestion and contribute to skin disorders such as eczema and acne.

In conclusion, Viruddha Ahara plays a significant role in the development and management of skin disorders according to Ayurveda. By avoiding incompatible food combinations, adopting balanced eating habits, and prioritizing nutrient-dense whole foods, individuals can support digestive health and maintain radiant skin. Ayurvedic principles offer valuable insights into the relationship between diet and skin health, guiding us towards holistic well-being.

Diagnosis of Skin Disorders According to Modern Medicine

Diagnosing skin disorders in modern medicine involves a meticulous process that combines medical history, physical examination, and sometimes additional diagnostic tests.

Introduction: Skin disorders affect millions worldwide, presenting a diverse array of symptoms and causes. Modern medicine employs a systematic approach to diagnose these conditions, ensuring accurate identification and tailored treatment plans.

Medical History: The diagnostic process typically begins with a comprehensive medical history. Patients are asked about their symptoms, their onset, duration, and any factors that exacerbate or alleviate them. Additionally, information regarding past medical conditions, medications, allergies, and family history of skin disorders is gathered. This step helps physicians narrow down potential diagnoses and understand the context of the patient's condition.

Physical Examination: A thorough physical examination of the skin is crucial for identifying visible signs of dermatological conditions. Physicians assess the color, texture, temperature, and moisture of the skin, as well as the presence of lesions, rashes, bumps, or other abnormalities. They may use a dermatoscope—a handheld device with magnification and light—to examine lesions more closely. This step allows for the visualization of characteristic patterns, helping in the differential diagnosis.

Diagnostic Tests: In some cases, additional diagnostic tests may be necessary to confirm or further investigate a suspected skin disorder. These tests can include:

Skin Biopsy: A small sample of skin tissue is collected and examined under a microscope to identify cellular abnormalities, inflammation, infections, or malignancies.
Patch Testing: Used to diagnose allergic contact dermatitis, patch testing involves applying small amounts of potential allergens to the skin to identify specific triggers.

Blood Tests: Blood tests may be ordered to assess levels of specific antibodies, detect infections, or evaluate systemic conditions that can manifest as skin disorders, such as autoimmune diseases.

Culture or Swab Tests: These tests involve collecting samples from skin lesions to identify the presence of bacteria, fungi, or viruses, aiding in the diagnosis of infectious skin conditions.

Specialized Imaging Techniques: In certain cases, specialized imaging techniques may be employed to visualize deeper skin structures or assess the extent of involvement. These can include:

Dermoscopy: This non-invasive imaging technique allows for the examination of skin lesions with enhanced visualization of surface structures and pigment patterns, aiding in the diagnosis of melanoma and other pigmented lesions.

Ultrasound: Ultrasound imaging can be used to evaluate the thickness of skin layers, identify fluid collections, or assess underlying structures such as muscles, tendons, or blood vessels.

Mri or Ct Scans: In rare or complex cases, magnetic resonance imaging (MRI) or computed tomography (CT) scans may be utilized to provide detailed images of the skin and underlying tissues, assisting in the diagnosis of deep-seated infections, tumors, or inflammatory conditions.

Conclusion: Diagnosing skin disorders in modern medicine is a multifaceted process that combines clinical evaluation, diagnostic tests, and sometimes specialized imaging techniques. By employing a systematic approach that integrates medical history, physical examination, and laboratory investigations, physicians can accurately identify skin conditions and develop personalized treatment strategies tailored to each patient's needs. Early and accurate diagnosis is essential for effective management and improved outcomes in individuals affected by dermatological disorders.

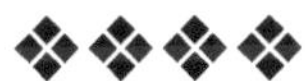

Chapter 4

MODALITIES USED IN SKIN DISORDERS

Skin disorders have been a prevalent concern throughout history, affecting millions worldwide. Both Ayurveda and modern medicine offer distinct approaches to understanding and treating these conditions.

According to Ayurveda

Ayurveda views skin disorders as manifestations of imbalances in the body's doshas (Vata, Pitta, and Kapha) and impurities in the blood (Rakta). Ayurvedic treatments focus on restoring balance and purifying the body through holistic approaches. Modalities include:

Herbal Remedies: Ayurvedic formulations often contain herbs like neem, turmeric, aloe vera, and manjistha, known for their anti-inflammatory, antimicrobial, and skin-soothing properties.

Dietary Changes: Ayurveda emphasizes dietary modifications to pacify aggravated doshas. For instance, Pitta-pacifying foods like cooling fruits and vegetables are recommended for Pitta-related skin disorders such as acne.

Panchakarma: This Ayurvedic detoxification therapy involves five cleansing procedures to eliminate toxins and restore balance. Vamana (emesis) and Virechana (purgation) are particularly beneficial for skin disorders by expelling accumulated toxins.

Lifestyle Modifications: Ayurveda stresses the importance of lifestyle factors such as stress management, adequate sleep, and regular exercise to maintain overall health, which indirectly impacts skin health.

According To Modern Medicine

Modern medicine adopts a scientific approach to diagnose and treat skin disorders, focusing on symptom relief and addressing underlying causes. Modalities commonly used in dermatology include:

Topical Treatments: Corticosteroids, retinoids, and antimicrobial agents are commonly prescribed to manage symptoms like inflammation, itching, and infection.

Systemic Medications: Oral medications such as antibiotics, antifungals, and immunosuppressants are prescribed for severe or widespread skin conditions like psoriasis and eczema.

Phototherapy: Light-based treatments like UVB phototherapy and PUVA therapy are used to target specific skin cells and reduce inflammation in conditions like psoriasis and vitiligo.

Laser Therapy: Various laser and light-based devices are employed to treat skin disorders by targeting specific structures or pigments, such as in the case of laser hair removal or scar reduction.

Comparison: While both Ayurveda and modern medicine aim to alleviate skin disorders, they differ in their philosophical foundations, diagnostic methods, and treatment approaches.

Ayurveda focuses on restoring balance within the body through holistic therapies, considering individual constitution and lifestyle factors, whereas modern medicine relies on standardized diagnostic procedures and evidence-based treatments.

Ayurvedic treatments may take longer to show results as they address underlying imbalances, while modern medicine often provides quicker symptom relief through targeted therapies.

Ayurvedic treatments are generally considered safer with fewer side effects, but their efficacy may vary based on individual responsiveness and adherence to lifestyle changes.

Modern medicine offers advanced technologies and pharmaceuticals for precise diagnosis and treatment, but these interventions may come with potential side effects and long-term risks.

Conclusion: Both Ayurveda and modern medicine offer valuable modalities for managing skin disorders, each with its own strengths and limitations. Integrating elements of both systems can provide comprehensive care, addressing the root causes of skin conditions while managing symptoms effectively. Collaborative efforts between Ayurvedic practitioners and dermatologists can enhance patient outcomes and promote holistic well-being.

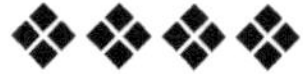

TREATMENT OF SKIN DISORDERS

ACNE VULGARIS (युवान पीडिका)

Acne Vulgaris According to Ayurveda

Acne vulgaris, known as युवान पीडिका in Ayurveda, is a common skin condition characterized by the formation of pimples, blackheads, whiteheads, and in severe cases, cysts. According to Ayurveda, acne is primarily caused by an imbalance in the body's doshas, primarily Pitta and Kapha.

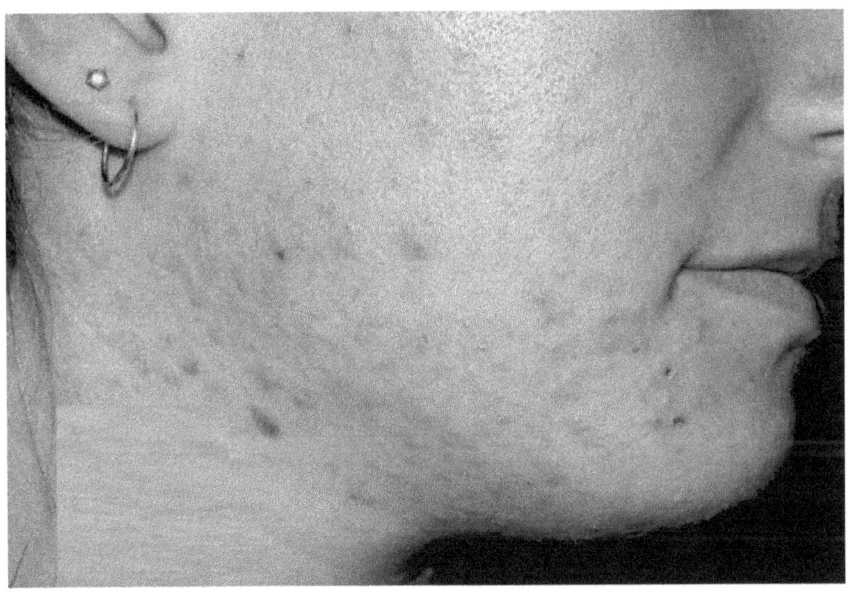

Dosha Imbalance: Ayurveda views acne as a result of aggravated Pitta and Kapha doshas. Pitta governs digestion and metabolism, while Kapha controls oil production and moisture balance in the body. When these doshas are imbalanced, impurities (ama) accumulate in the body, leading to the manifestation of acne.

Diet and Lifestyle Factors: According to Ayurveda, dietary habits and lifestyle choices play a crucial role in the development of acne. Consuming excessive spicy, oily, and fried foods aggravates Pitta dosha, leading to inflammation and the formation of acne. Irregular eating habits, excessive consumption of caffeine and alcohol, and inadequate sleep also contribute to dosha imbalance and acne.

Poor Digestion: Weak digestion (agni) is considered a significant factor in the development of acne in Ayurveda. When digestion is impaired, toxins (ama) are not properly eliminated from the body, leading to the accumulation of impurities in the skin and the manifestation of acne.

Hormonal Imbalance: In Ayurveda, hormonal imbalance is often attributed to the aggravation of Pitta dosha, leading to increased sebum production and inflammation in the skin. This imbalance can be triggered by factors such as stress, menstrual irregularities, and hormonal fluctuations during puberty.

Herbal Remedies: Ayurveda offers a variety of herbal remedies for treating acne vulgaris. These remedies focus on pacifying Pitta and Kapha doshas, improving digestion, and purifying the blood. Some commonly used herbs include neem, turmeric, aloe vera, sandalwood, and manjistha. These herbs can be used both internally and externally in the form of powders, pastes, decoctions, and oils.

Dietary Recommendations: Ayurveda emphasizes the importance of a balanced diet in managing acne vulgaris. Foods that are cooling, hydrating, and easy to digest are recommended to pacify Pitta and Kapha doshas. This includes fresh fruits and vegetables, whole grains, legumes, and plenty of water. Avoiding spicy, oily, and processed foods is essential to prevent further aggravation of acne.

Lifestyle Modifications: In addition to dietary changes, Ayurveda suggests adopting a healthy lifestyle to manage acne vulgaris. Regular exercise, stress management techniques such as yoga and meditation, adequate sleep, and maintaining proper hygiene are essential for balancing the doshas and promoting clear, radiant skin.

In conclusion, Ayurveda offers a holistic approach to managing acne vulgaris by addressing the root cause of the condition through dosha balancing, dietary modifications, herbal remedies, and lifestyle interventions. By adopting these principles, individuals can effectively manage acne and promote overall skin health.

Acne Vulgaris in Modern Medicine

Acne vulgaris is a common skin condition in modern medicine characterized by the formation of pimples, blackheads, whiteheads, and in severe cases, cysts. It primarily affects areas of the skin with a high concentration of oil glands, such as the face, chest, and back. Let's explore acne vulgaris from the perspective of modern medicine:

Pathophysiology: Acne vulgaris is primarily caused by several factors, including excess sebum production, clogged hair follicles, bacterial overgrowth (Propionibacterium acnes), and inflammation. Hormonal changes, particularly during puberty, pregnancy, and menstruation, can also contribute to the development of acne.

TYPES OF ACNE: ONES): Non-Inflammatory (COMEDONES): lesions consisting of open comedones (blackheads) and closed comedones (whiteheads).

Inflammatory Lesions: These include papules, pustules, nodules, and cysts, which result from inflammation of the hair follicles due to bacterial infection.

Treatment Approaches: Modern medicine offers several treatment options for acne vulgaris, depending on the severity and type of lesions:

Topical Treatments: These include over-the-counter and prescription medications containing ingredients such as benzoyl peroxide, salicylic acid, retinoids, and antibiotics to reduce inflammation, unclog pores, and kill bacteria.

Oral Medications: In cases of moderate to severe acne, oral antibiotics, oral contraceptives (for females), and oral retinoids (isotretinoin) may be prescribed to target bacteria, reduce sebum production, and regulate hormonal imbalances.

Procedures: Dermatological procedures such as chemical peels, microdermabrasion, laser therapy, and extraction of comedones may be recommended for stubborn or severe cases of acne.

Prevention and Lifestyle Modifications: Preventive measures and lifestyle modifications can help manage acne vulgaris:

Daily Skincare Routine: Gentle cleansing with non-comedogenic products, avoiding harsh scrubbing, and using oil-free moisturizers can help prevent the worsening of acne.

Dietary Considerations: While diet alone may not directly cause acne, some individuals may find that certain foods, such as dairy and high-glycemic-index foods, exacerbate their symptoms. Maintaining a balanced diet rich in fruits, vegetables, whole grains, and lean proteins may support overall skin health.

Stress Management: Stress can exacerbate acne through hormonal fluctuations. Practicing stress-reducing techniques such as mindfulness, meditation, and regular exercise may help manage acne symptoms.

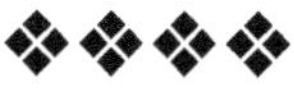

ALOPECIA AREATA (इन्द्रलुप्त)

Alopecia Areata According to Ayurveda

Alopecia areata, a condition characterized by hair loss in patches, is a complex issue often addressed through various medical perspectives, including Ayurveda. According to Ayurvedic principles, alopecia areata is primarily caused by imbalances in the body's doshas, particularly Pitta and Vata doshas, along with impaired digestion and accumulation of toxins (ama) in the body.

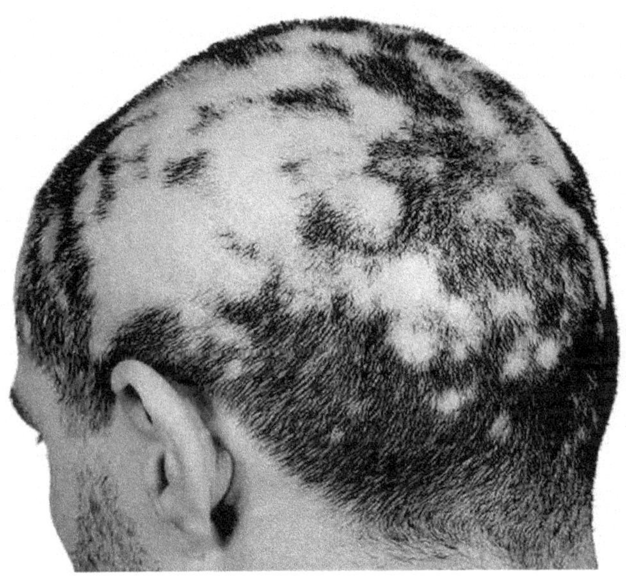

In Ayurveda, alopecia areata is classified under the category of siraja-unmada (mental disorders with physical symptoms), as it affects both physical appearance and mental well-being. The condition is often associated with excess Pitta dosha, leading to inflammation and overheating of the scalp. Additionally, imbalances in Vata dosha can disrupt the hair follicles' nourishment and contribute to hair loss.

Ayurvedic treatment for alopecia areata aims to balance the doshas, purify the body, and rejuvenate the scalp and hair follicles. Here are some key components of Ayurvedic management for alopecia areata:

Dietary Modifications: Ayurveda emphasizes the importance of a balanced diet to maintain overall health and balance the doshas. Individuals with alopecia areata are advised to avoid Pitta-aggravating foods such as spicy, fried, and acidic foods. Instead, they should consume cooling and nourishing foods like fresh fruits, vegetables, whole grains, and dairy products.

Herbal Remedies: Ayurvedic herbs are used to pacify Pitta and Vata doshas, improve digestion, and detoxify the body. Some commonly prescribed herbs for alopecia areata include Bhringraj (Eclipta alba), Amla (Indian gooseberry), Brahmi (Bacopa monnieri), Neem (Azadirachta indica), and Ashwagandha (Withania somnifera).

Ayurvedic Therapies: Various therapies are employed to stimulate hair growth, promote scalp health, and reduce stress, which is considered a significant factor in aggravating Pitta dosha. These therapies may include Shirodhara (pouring of medicated oil on the forehead), Nasya (nasal administration of medicated oils), Abhyanga (therapeutic oil massage), and Panchakarma (detoxification procedures).

Lifestyle Modifications: Ayurveda emphasizes the importance of a healthy lifestyle to maintain balance and prevent disease. Individuals with alopecia areata are advised to manage stress through practices like yoga, meditation, and pranayama (breathing exercises). Adequate sleep and regular exercise are also essential for overall well-being.

Customized Treatment Plans: Ayurvedic practitioners tailor treatment plans according to the individual's constitution (Prakriti), imbalances (Vikriti), and specific symptoms. The treatment may involve a combination of dietary recommendations, herbal supplements, lifestyle modifications, and therapeutic interventions.

It's important to note that Ayurvedic treatment for alopecia areata may take time to show results, as it focuses on addressing the root cause of the condition rather than just alleviating symptoms.

Alopecia Areata in Modern Medicine

In modern medicine, alopecia areata is considered an autoimmune disorder, where the body's immune system mistakenly attacks the hair follicles, leading to hair loss.

Autoimmune Mechanism: In alopecia areata, the immune system targets the hair follicles, mistakenly recognizing them as foreign invaders. This immune attack disrupts the normal hair growth cycle, leading to hair loss. The exact cause of this autoimmune response is not fully understood, but genetic factors, environmental triggers, and alterations in immune function are believed to play a role.

Symptoms: Alopecia areata typically presents as round or oval patches of hair loss on the scalp or other hair-bearing areas of the body. In some cases, the condition may progress to total scalp hair loss (alopecia totalis) or complete body hair loss (alopecia universalis). Hair loss in alopecia areata is usually non-scarring, meaning the hair follicles remain intact and have the potential to regrow hair.

Diagnosis: Diagnosis of alopecia areata is usually based on a physical examination and medical history. In some cases, a scalp biopsy may be performed to confirm the diagnosis and rule out other conditions that cause hair loss. Dermatologists are the primary healthcare providers who diagnose and manage alopecia areata.

Treatment Options: Treatment for alopecia areata aims to suppress the autoimmune response, stimulate hair regrowth, and manage associated symptoms. Common treatment options include:

Corticosteroids: Topical or injected corticosteroids are often used to reduce inflammation and suppress the immune response in the affected areas.

Minoxidil: Topical minoxidil, a medication that promotes hair growth, may be prescribed to encourage regrowth in affected areas.

Immunotherapy: Agents such as diphencyprone (DPCP) or squaric acid dibutyl ester (SADBE) are applied to the skin to induce an allergic reaction, which may stimulate hair regrowth.

Jak Inhibitors: Janus kinase (JAK) inhibitors, such as tofacitinib and ruxolitinib, are oral medications that suppress the immune response and have shown promise in treating alopecia areata in clinical trials.

Psychosocial Impact: Hair loss, especially when it occurs suddenly and unpredictably, can have significant psychosocial effects on individuals with alopecia areata. Support groups, counseling, and psychotherapy may be beneficial in addressing the emotional impact of the condition and helping individuals cope with their hair loss.

Prognosis: The prognosis for alopecia areata varies among individuals. In some cases, spontaneous hair regrowth may occur without treatment, while others may experience recurrent episodes of hair loss. The effectiveness of treatment also varies, and some individuals may not respond to conventional therapies.

Overall, alopecia areata is a complex condition with multiple underlying factors, and treatment approaches in modern medicine focus on managing the autoimmune response and promoting hair regrowth while addressing the psychosocial impact of the condition.

BED SORES (शैय्या व्रण)

Bed Sores According to Ayurveda

Bed sores, also known as pressure ulcers or decubitus ulcers, are a significant concern in healthcare, particularly for individuals with limited mobility or who are bedridden. Bed sores primarily occur due to prolonged pressure on the skin and tissues, leading to impaired blood circulation and tissue damage.

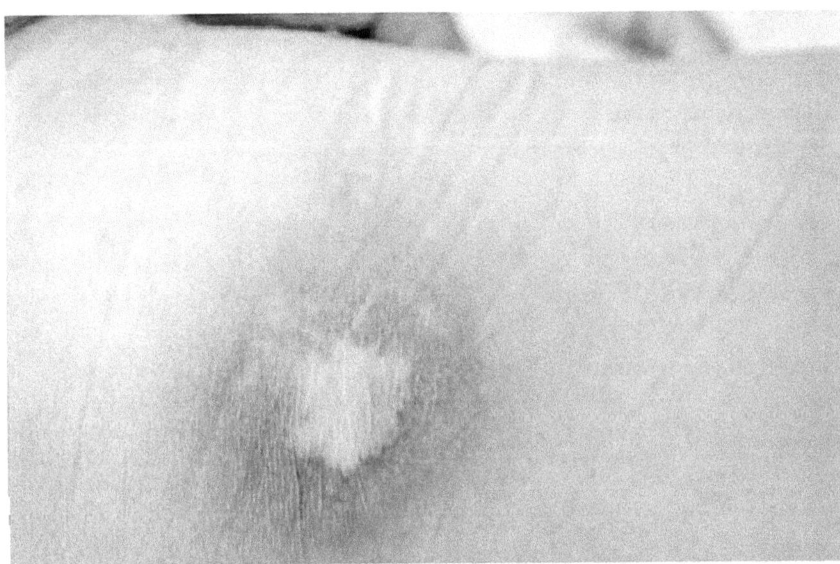

Causes According to Ayurveda:

Vata Imbalance: Ayurveda identifies Vata dosha as the primary culprit behind bed sores. When Vata becomes aggravated, it causes dryness, roughness, and constriction in the affected area, impairing the nourishment and oxygenation of tissues.

Poor Nutrition: According to Ayurveda, inadequate nutrition can exacerbate Vata imbalance, leading to weakened tissues and increased susceptibility to bed sores.

Immobility: Prolonged immobility leads to stagnation of Vata and aggravates its qualities, predisposing individuals to bed sores.

Dehydration: Dehydration contributes to dryness in the body, worsening Vata imbalance and making the skin more susceptible to damage.

Symptoms in Ayurveda:

Dryness and Roughness: The affected skin becomes dry, rough, and prone to cracking due to aggravated Vata.

Discoloration: Ayurveda recognizes changes in skin color as indicative of underlying doshic imbalances. In the case of bed sores, the affected area may appear darker or discolored.

Pain and Sensitivity: As the condition progresses, individuals may experience pain, tenderness, or sensitivity in the affected area, reflecting the aggravation of Vata dosha.

Ayurvedic Management of Bed Sores

Balancing Vata Dosha: The primary goal of Ayurvedic treatment for bed sores is to pacify aggravated Vata dosha. This involves adopting a Vata-pacifying diet and lifestyle, including warm, nourishing foods, adequate hydration, and gentle, regular movement to prevent stagnation.

External Applications: Ayurveda advocates the use of herbal oils and pastes for external application to nourish and moisturize the affected skin, promote healing, and prevent further damage. Oils such as sesame oil infused with herbs like neem, turmeric, or ashwagandha are commonly used for this purpose.

Herbal Remedies: Internal herbal remedies may also be prescribed to address underlying imbalances and support tissue regeneration. Herbs with moisturizing, anti-inflammatory, and rejuvenating properties, such as ashwagandha, guduchi, and shatavari, are often recommended in Ayurvedic formulations for bed sores.

Wound Care: Proper wound care is essential in Ayurveda to prevent infection and promote healing. This includes keeping the affected area clean, using natural antiseptics such as turmeric or honey, and covering the wound with clean, breathable dressings.

Preventive Measures:

Regular Repositioning: Ayurveda emphasizes the importance of regular movement to prevent stagnation and alleviate pressure on vulnerable areas. Caregivers should assist bedridden individuals in changing positions frequently to reduce the risk of bed sores.

Optimal Nutrition: A balanced diet rich in nutrients is crucial for maintaining healthy skin and tissues. Ayurveda recommends foods that are nourishing, easy to digest, and supportive of overall well-being.

Hydration: Adequate hydration is essential for maintaining skin health and preventing dryness. Ayurveda advises drinking warm fluids and herbal teas to keep the body hydrated and balanced.

Bed Sores in Modern Medicine

In modern medicine, bed sores, also known as pressure ulcers, are a significant concern, particularly for individuals with limited mobility or who spend extended periods in bed or seated. These ulcers develop when pressure on the skin and underlying tissues reduces blood flow to the area, leading to tissue damage and eventually ulceration.
Bed sores are categorized into four stages based on their severity, ranging from stage 1, which involves superficial redness and irritation, to stage 4, which involves deep tissue damage and potential necrosis (tissue death).

Causes in Modern Medicine:

Pressure: Prolonged pressure on the skin and soft tissues is the primary cause of bed sores. This pressure disrupts blood flow to the area, depriving tissues of oxygen and nutrients, leading to tissue damage.

Shear and Friction: Shear occurs when layers of tissue slide over each other, while friction occurs when the skin rubs against another surface. Both shear and friction can contribute to the development of bed sores, especially in combination with pressure.

Moisture: Excessive moisture from sweat, urine, or feces can soften the skin and make it more susceptible to damage. Moisture also contributes to bacterial growth, increasing the risk of infection in bed sores.

Poor Nutrition: Malnutrition or dehydration can impair the body's ability to repair damaged tissues, making individuals more vulnerable to developing bed sores.

Symptoms in Modern Medicine:

Skin Discoloration: In the early stages, bed sores may appear as areas of redness or discoloration on the skin, indicating tissue damage.

Skin Texture Changes: As the condition progresses, the affected skin may become warm, swollen, or tender to the touch. In severe cases, the skin may develop blisters or open wounds.

Pain or Discomfort: Individuals with bed sores may experience pain, itching, or discomfort in the affected area, particularly when pressure is applied.

Odor or Drainage: In advanced stages, bed sores may produce foul-smelling discharge or pus, indicating tissue breakdown and potential infection.

Modern Treatment Approaches:

Pressure Relief: The primary goal of treatment is to relieve pressure on affected areas to promote healing. This may involve repositioning patients regularly, using specialized support surfaces such as pressure-relieving mattresses or cushions, and minimizing pressure on vulnerable areas.

Wound Care: Proper wound care is essential for managing bed sores and preventing complications. This includes cleaning the wound with mild soap

and water, removing dead tissue (debridement), applying dressings to promote healing, and managing any underlying infections with antibiotics if necessary.

Nutritional Support: Adequate nutrition is crucial for wound healing and tissue repair. Patients with bed sores may require nutritional supplements or dietary modifications to ensure they receive sufficient protein, vitamins, and minerals to support healing.

Pain Management: Pain associated with bed sores can be managed with medications such as analgesics or topical treatments to alleviate discomfort and improve quality of life.

Preventive Measures:

Regular Skin Assessment: Healthcare providers should regularly assess patients' skin for signs of pressure ulcers and implement preventive measures as needed.

Mobility and Positioning: Encouraging mobility and changing positions frequently can help reduce pressure on vulnerable areas and prevent the development of bed sores.

Skin Care: Keeping the skin clean, dry, and well-moisturized can help prevent skin breakdown and reduce the risk of bed sores.

Education: Educating patients, caregivers, and healthcare providers about the risk factors and preventive measures for bed sores is essential for early detection and effective management.

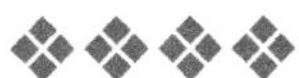

BOILS (फुंसी)

Boils According to Ayurveda

Boils, known as "फुंसी" in Ayurveda, are a common skin condition characterized by painful, pus-filled bumps that arise from infected hair follicles or oil glands. According to Ayurveda, boils are primarily caused by an imbalance in the body's doshas, particularly the pitta and kapha doshas.

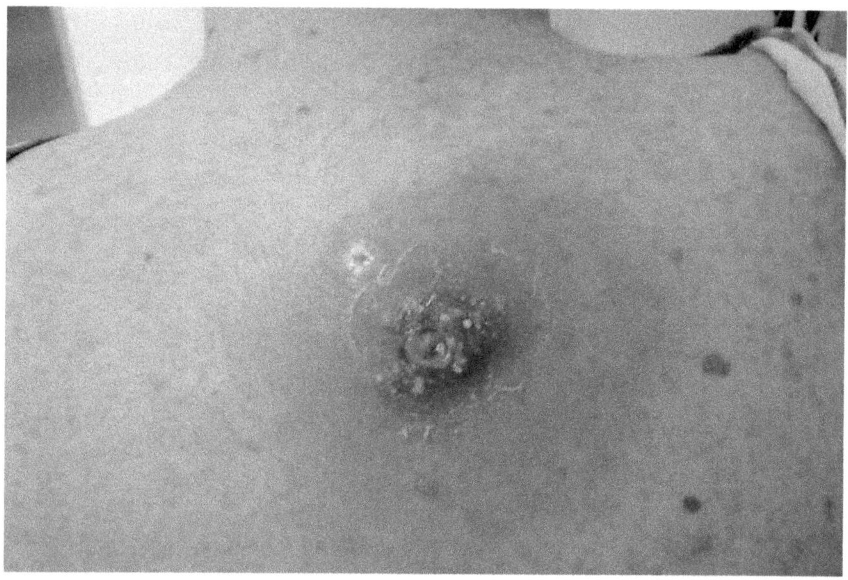

Boils are considered a manifestation of excess pitta dosha in the body. Pitta dosha governs metabolism, digestion, and transformation processes in the body. When pitta becomes aggravated due to factors like poor diet, excessive consumption of spicy or oily foods, stress, and poor hygiene, it can lead to the formation of boils. Additionally, an imbalance in kapha dosha, which governs lubrication and stability, can contribute to the accumulation of toxins in the body, further exacerbating the condition.

Ayurvedic remedies for boils aim to pacify aggravated pitta and kapha doshas while promoting detoxification and purification of the body. Here are some detailed approaches according to Ayurveda:

Dietary Modifications: Ayurveda emphasizes the importance of maintaining a balanced diet to prevent and manage boils. Individuals prone to boils should avoid spicy, oily, and processed foods that can aggravate pitta dosha. Instead, focus on a diet that is cooling, hydrating, and rich in fresh fruits, vegetables, whole grains, and legumes. Bitter and astringent foods like bitter gourd, neem, and leafy greens help detoxify the body and reduce inflammation.

Herbal Remedies: Ayurvedic herbs are instrumental in treating boils and balancing the doshas. Neem (Azadirachta indica), turmeric (Curcuma longa), and Aloe vera are renowned for their anti-inflammatory, antibacterial, and detoxifying properties. Neem and turmeric can be applied topically as a paste or taken internally to cleanse the blood and reduce inflammation. Aloe vera gel soothes irritated skin and promotes healing.

Detoxification Therapies: Panchakarma, the detoxification process in Ayurveda, is highly beneficial for individuals with recurrent boils. Procedures like Virechana (therapeutic purgation) and Raktamokshana (bloodletting) help eliminate toxins from the body, purify the blood, and alleviate inflammation. These therapies should be performed under the guidance of a qualified Ayurvedic practitioner.

Lifestyle Modifications: Stress management techniques such as yoga, meditation, and pranayama (breathwork) play a crucial role in managing boils. Stress can exacerbate pitta imbalance, leading to flare-ups of boils. Practicing relaxation techniques helps calm the mind, reduce stress hormones, and restore balance to the doshas.

Hygiene Practices: Maintaining good personal hygiene is essential for preventing the spread of infection and reducing the risk of boils. Ayurveda recommends daily self-massage (abhyanga) with cooling oils like coconut or neem oil to nourish the skin, improve circulation, and pacify aggravated doshas. Regular bathing with herbal decoctions or powders containing antimicrobial herbs like neem and turmeric can also help keep the skin clean and healthy.

Boils in Modern Medicine

Boils, known as "फुंसी" in Hindi, are a common skin condition in modern medicine as well. They are typically caused by a bacterial infection of hair follicles or oil glands, most commonly by Staphylococcus aureus bacteria. Here's a detailed essay on boils from the perspective of modern medicine:

Boils, medically termed as furuncles or abscesses, are painful, pus-filled bumps that develop on the skin. They often start as red, tender nodules and gradually become larger and more painful as they fill with pus. Boils can occur anywhere on the body but are most commonly found in areas where friction or sweating occurs, such as the face, neck, armpits, buttocks, and thighs.

The primary cause of boils is the entry of bacteria, usually Staphylococcus aureus, into the skin through cuts, breaks, or hair follicles. These bacteria multiply rapidly, causing an inflammatory response by the body's immune system, leading to the formation of a boil. Factors that increase the risk of developing boils include poor hygiene, compromised immune function, diabetes, obesity, and certain skin conditions such as eczema or acne.

The Typical Progression of a Boil Involves the Following Stages:

Infection: Bacteria enter the skin through a break or hair follicle, causing inflammation and infection.

Inflammation: The body's immune system responds to the infection, resulting in redness, swelling, and tenderness around the affected area.

Pus Formation: As the infection progresses, the body forms a pocket of pus (a mixture of dead white blood cells, bacteria, and tissue debris) within the skin, resulting in the characteristic appearance of a boil.

Maturation and Rupture: Over time, the boil continues to enlarge until it reaches a point where it may spontaneously rupture, draining pus and relieving pressure. In some cases, medical intervention such as incision and drainage may be necessary to facilitate drainage and promote healing.

Treatment for Boils in Modern Medicine Typically Involves:

Warm Compresses: Applying warm compresses to the affected area helps to increase blood circulation, reduce pain, and promote spontaneous drainage of the boil.

Antibiotics: In cases of severe or recurrent boils, oral or topical antibiotics may be prescribed to eliminate the bacterial infection and prevent further complications.

Incision and Drainage: If a boil does not respond to conservative treatment or becomes extremely painful, a healthcare provider may perform a minor surgical procedure to make an incision and drain the pus from the boil.

PainManagement: Over-the-counter pain relievers such as acetaminophen or ibuprofen may be recommended to alleviate pain and discomfort associated with boils.

Preventive Measures: Practicing good hygiene, including regular handwashing, keeping skin clean and dry, and avoiding sharing personal items such as towels or razors, can help prevent the spread of bacteria and reduce the risk of developing boils.

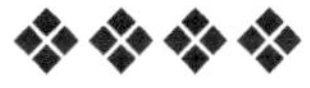

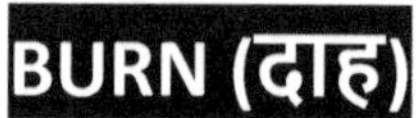

BURN (दाह)

Burn According to Ayurveda

In Ayurveda, burn injuries, known as "Daha" are classified based on various factors such as the cause, severity, and dosha involvement. Ayurveda offers a holistic approach to manage burns, focusing on alleviating pain, preventing infections, promoting wound healing, and minimizing scarring.

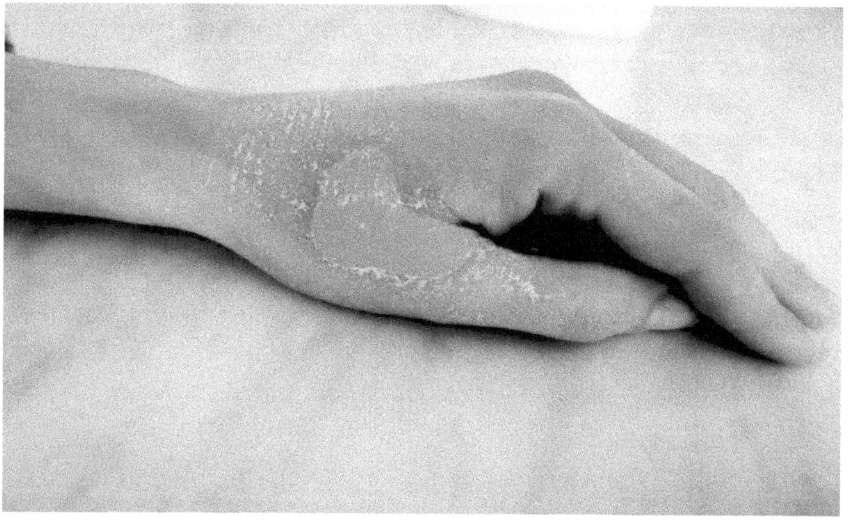

Classification of Burns: Ayurveda classifies burns based on the causative factors and dosha involvement:

Vataja Daha: Burns caused by exposure to dry heat or wind, characterized by symptoms such as dryness, pain, and roughness.

Pittaja Daha: Burns resulting from exposure to heat or fire, associated with symptoms like inflammation, redness, and intense burning sensation.

Kaphaja Daha: Burns caused by exposure to cold or moist heat, leading to symptoms like swelling, oozing, and heaviness.

Pathophysiology of Burns: According to Ayurveda, burns disrupt the balance of the doshas (Vata, Pitta, and Kapha) and vital energies (prana, tejas, and ojas) in the body. The aggravated doshas manifest as various symptoms depending on the type and severity of the burn.

Clinical Presentation: The clinical presentation of burns in Ayurveda includes symptoms such as pain, inflammation, blistering, redness, swelling, and impaired skin integrity. In severe cases, burns can lead to complications like infection, fluid loss, shock, and scarring.

Ayurvedic Management of Burns: Ayurvedic treatment aims to restore the balance of the doshas, promote tissue regeneration, and prevent complications. The management of burns involves the following approaches:

Cooling Therapies: Application of cooling substances like aloe vera gel, sandalwood paste, coconut oil, or cucumber juice to soothe the burning sensation and reduce inflammation.

Herbal Remedies: Administration of herbal formulations containing ingredients like turmeric, neem, manjistha, and licorice to promote wound healing, prevent infection, and reduce inflammation.

Oil Therapy: Application of medicated oils such as coconut oil, sesame oil, or ghee infused with herbs like turmeric, neem, or Brahmi to nourish the skin, alleviate pain, and promote tissue repair.

Panchakarma: Ayurvedic detoxification therapies like Virechana (purgation) or Raktamokshana (bloodletting) may be recommended to eliminate toxins and purify the blood, thereby facilitating healing.

Dietary Recommendations: Consumption of cooling and hydrating foods like fresh fruits, vegetables, and herbal teas to support the body's healing process and replenish lost fluids.

Lifestyle Modifications: Avoidance of exposure to extreme temperatures, wearing protective clothing, and practicing stress-reducing techniques like yoga and meditation to promote overall well-being.

Burn in Modern Medicine

In modern medicine, burns are classified based on the depth and severity of tissue damage, ranging from first-degree to fourth-degree burns. Here's an essay outlining burn injuries in modern medicine:

Burn injuries are common occurrences that result from exposure to heat, chemicals, electricity, or radiation. In modern medicine, burns are classified based on their depth, extent, and severity, and they require prompt assessment and appropriate management to prevent complications and promote healing.

Classification of Burns: Modern medicine categorizes burns into four main types:

First-Degree Burns: These affect only the outer layer of the skin (epidermis), causing redness, pain, and mild swelling. Sunburns are common examples of first-degree burns.

Second-Degree Burns: These damage the epidermis and part of the underlying layer (dermis), leading to blistering, severe pain, redness, and swelling. These burns may also appear wet or weepy.

Third-Degree Burns: These destroy the entire thickness of the skin, extending into the deeper tissues. They are characterized by white or charred appearance, numbness, and potential damage to nerves, blood vessels, and muscles.

Fourth-Degree Burns: These are the most severe and extend beyond the skin into the underlying fat, muscles, or bones. They often result in blackened, charred, or carbonized tissue and require extensive medical intervention.

Pathophysiology of Burns: Burn injuries disrupt the skin's barrier function and lead to a cascade of inflammatory responses, including increased vascular permeability, fluid loss, and tissue damage. Severe burns can also trigger systemic effects such as hypovolemia, electrolyte imbalances, and compromised immune function.

Clinical Presentation: The clinical presentation of burns varies depending on the type and severity but commonly includes symptoms such as pain, redness, swelling, blistering, charred skin, and impaired tissue integrity. In severe cases, burns can lead to shock, respiratory distress, and multiorgan dysfunction.

Modern Management of Burns: The management of burns in modern medicine involves the following strategies:

Assessment and Stabilization: Prompt assessment of burn depth and extent, followed by stabilization of vital signs and initiation of fluid resuscitation to prevent hypovolemic shock.

Wound Care: Depending on the severity, wound care may involve cleaning, debridement, and application of topical antimicrobial agents or specialized dressings to prevent infection and promote healing.

Pain Management: Administration of analgesic medications to alleviate pain and discomfort associated with burns, including nonsteroidal anti-inflammatory drugs (NSAIDs), opioids, and topical anesthetics.

Fluid Resuscitation: Calculation and administration of intravenous fluids to maintain adequate hydration, replace fluid losses, and support organ perfusion.

Surgical Interventions: Surgical procedures such as skin grafting, debridement, and escharotomy may be necessary for deep or extensive burns to remove damaged tissue, restore skin integrity, and improve functional outcomes.

Nutritional Support: Provision of adequate nutrition and supplementation to meet increased metabolic demands and support tissue repair and regeneration.

Rehabilitation: physical therapy, occupational therapy, and psychological support to optimize functional recovery, prevent contractures, and address psychosocial issues associated with burn injuries.

❖ ❖ ❖ ❖

CANDIDIASIS (कैंडिडिआसिस)

Candidiasis in Ayurveda

Candidiasis, known as "कैंडिडिआसिस" in Ayurveda, is a condition caused by an overgrowth of the Candida fungus, primarily Candida albicans, in the body. In Ayurveda, it is classified under the category of "Kushta" or skin disorders. The ancient texts of Ayurveda, such as Charaka Samhita and Sushruta Samhita, describe Candidiasis as a result of an imbalance in the body's doshas, mainly Pitta and Kapha.

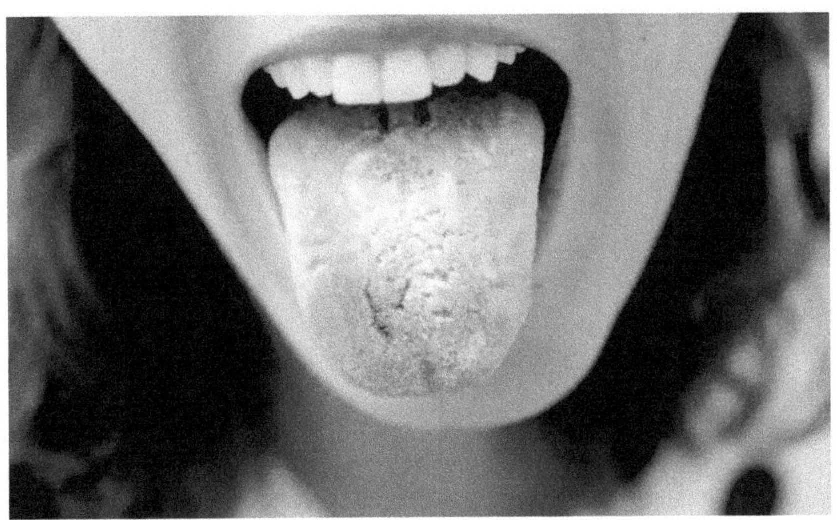

According to Ayurveda, Candidiasis occurs when there is an accumulation of ama (toxins) in the body due to poor digestion and weak immune function. This ama, along with aggravated Pitta and Kapha doshas, creates an environment conducive to the growth of Candida fungus, leading to various symptoms such as itching, burning sensation, redness, and discharge in affected areas like the mouth, genitalia, and skin folds.

Treatment in Ayurveda focuses on restoring the balance of doshas, eliminating toxins, and strengthening the immune system. This is achieved through a combination of dietary changes, lifestyle modifications, herbal remedies, and cleansing procedures known as Panchakarma.

Dietary Modifications: Ayurveda emphasizes a diet that pacifies Pitta and Kapha doshas while improving digestion. This includes avoiding spicy, oily, and sugary foods, and incorporating cooling, bitter, and astringent tastes. Fresh fruits, vegetables, whole grains, and herbs like neem, turmeric, and aloe vera are recommended.

Lifestyle Changes: Stress management techniques such as yoga, meditation, and pranayama (breathing exercises) are essential to reduce Pitta aggravation. Adequate sleep and regular exercise also play a crucial role in boosting immunity and maintaining overall health.

Herbal Remedies: Ayurvedic herbs with anti-fungal, anti-inflammatory, and immune-stimulating properties are used to combat Candidiasis. Some commonly prescribed herbs include neem, turmeric, triphala, guduchi, and kutki. These herbs can be consumed internally as decoctions, powders, or tablets, and applied topically as pastes or oils.

Panchakarma Therapies: Panchakarma, the Ayurvedic detoxification and rejuvenation therapy, helps to eliminate ama and balance the doshas. Therapies such as Vamana (emesis), Virechana (purgation), and Basti (enema) are tailored to the individual's constitution and condition to remove toxins from the body.

Hygiene Practices: Maintaining proper hygiene is crucial in preventing the spread and recurrence of Candidiasis. This includes keeping the affected areas clean and dry, wearing loose-fitting clothes made of breathable fabrics, and avoiding excessive use of antibiotics and corticosteroids.

In conclusion, Ayurveda offers a holistic approach to managing Candidiasis by addressing the root cause of the imbalance in the body's constitution and promoting overall health and well-being through diet, lifestyle, herbal remedies, and detoxification therapies. However, it's essential to consult with a qualified Ayurvedic practitioner for personalized treatment based on individual needs and constitution.

Candidiasis in Modern Medicine

In modern medicine, Candidiasis is a fungal infection caused by Candida species, primarily Candida albicans. It can manifest in various forms, including oral thrush, vaginal yeast infections, and systemic candidiasis, depending on the affected area and the severity of the infection.

Risk Factors: Certain factors increase the risk of Candidiasis, such as weakened immune system (due to conditions like HIV/AIDS or cancer), diabetes, pregnancy, use of antibiotics or corticosteroids, and lifestyle factors like poor hygiene and wearing tight clothing.

Symptoms: The symptoms of Candidiasis vary depending on the affected area but commonly include itching, burning sensation, redness, swelling, and discharge. In systemic candidiasis, symptoms may include fever, chills, and fatigue, indicating a more severe infection affecting internal organs.

Diagnosis: Diagnosis of Candidiasis typically involves a physical examination and may include laboratory tests such as culture or microscopy of the affected area to confirm the presence of Candida fungus. In systemic candidiasis, blood cultures and imaging tests may be performed to assess the extent of the infection.

Treatment: Treatment of Candidiasis in modern medicine usually involves antifungal medications, both topical and systemic, depending on the severity and location of the infection. Common antifungal agents include fluconazole, clotrimazole, miconazole, and nystatin. In severe cases or systemic infections, intravenous antifungal medications may be necessary.

Prevention: Preventive measures for Candidiasis include practicing good hygiene, maintaining a healthy diet, avoiding unnecessary use of antibiotics and corticosteroids, wearing loose-fitting clothing made of breathable fabrics, and managing underlying medical conditions such as diabetes or immunodeficiency.

Complications: If left untreated, Candidiasis can lead to complications such as recurrent infections, spread to other parts of the body (especially in immunocompromised individuals), and systemic candidiasis can result in serious complications such as septicemia or organ failure.

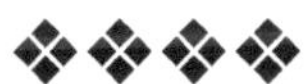

CARBUNCLES (शतपोनक)

Carbuncles in Ayurveda

Carbuncles, known as "शतपोनक" in Ayurveda, are a significant health concern addressed in ancient Ayurvedic texts. In Ayurveda, carbuncles are understood as a manifestation of imbalanced doshas, primarily Pitta and Kapha. Pitta, representing fire and water elements, governs metabolism and digestion, while Kapha, associated with earth and water elements, regulates structure and lubrication in the body.

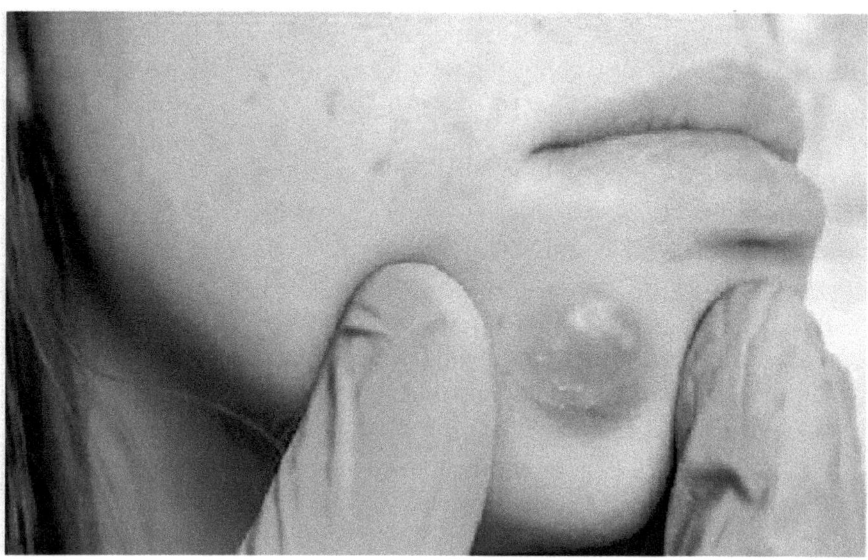

According to Ayurvedic principles, the formation of carbuncles is attributed to the accumulation of toxins, known as "ama," within the body, which disrupts the equilibrium of doshas. This accumulation can occur due to poor dietary habits, sedentary lifestyle, inadequate digestion, or environmental factors.

Carbuncles are characterized by the formation of deep-seated, painful, and inflamed clusters of boils on the skin, often accompanied by fever and general malaise. Ayurvedic texts emphasize the importance of addressing the root cause of carbuncles by rebalancing the doshas and eliminating the accumulated toxins from the body.

Treatment in Ayurveda typically involves a holistic approach that includes dietary modifications, lifestyle changes, herbal remedies, and therapeutic procedures. Here are some key aspects of managing carbuncles according to Ayurveda:

Pitta-Pacifying Diet: To alleviate symptoms and rebalance Pitta dosha, individuals are advised to consume cooling and hydrating foods such as fresh fruits, vegetables, whole grains, and herbal teas. Spicy, fried, and processed foods should be avoided as they can aggravate Pitta.

Detoxification: Ayurveda emphasizes detoxification therapies, known as "Panchakarma," to eliminate ama from the body. These therapies include techniques such as herbal steam therapy (Swedana), purgation (Virechana), and bloodletting (Raktamokshana), which help in cleansing the body and restoring doshic balance.

Herbal Remedies: Various Ayurvedic herbs are known for their detoxifying, anti-inflammatory, and antimicrobial properties, which can aid in the management of carbuncles. Examples include neem (Azadirachta indica), turmeric (Curcuma longa), manjistha (Rubia cordifolia), and guduchi (Tinospora cordifolia). These herbs can be consumed internally or applied topically as pastes or oils.

External Therapies: Localized treatments such as poultices, herbal compresses, and medicated oils can help alleviate pain, reduce inflammation, and promote healing of carbuncles. Ayurvedic oils infused with herbs like neem, turmeric, and manjistha are commonly used for topical application.

Lifestyle Recommendations: Ayurveda emphasizes the importance of maintaining a balanced lifestyle to prevent the recurrence of carbuncles. This includes practicing stress-reducing techniques, getting adequate rest, engaging in regular physical activity, and maintaining personal hygiene.

Carbuncle in Modern Medicine

In modern medicine, a carbuncle is referred to as a cluster of connected furuncles (boils) that occur beneath the skin. It's typically caused by a bacterial infection, most commonly Staphylococcus aureus. Carbuncles often develop in areas with hair follicles, such as the back of the neck, thighs, or shoulders.

The symptoms of carbuncles include red, swollen, and painful skin lesions that may contain pus. Other symptoms can include fever, fatigue, and general malaise.

Treatment for carbuncles in modern medicine usually involves:

Antibiotics: Oral or topical antibiotics are often prescribed to treat the bacterial infection and prevent its spread. Depending on the severity of the infection, antibiotics may be taken for a week or longer.

Incision and Drainage: In some cases, especially when the carbuncle is large or does not respond to antibiotics, a healthcare professional may need to make an incision to drain the pus and relieve pressure. This procedure is typically done under local anesthesia.

Warm Compresses: Applying warm compresses to the affected area can help reduce pain and promote drainage of the carbuncle. This can be done several times a day.

Pain Relief: Over-the-counter pain relievers such as ibuprofen or acetaminophen may be recommended to alleviate discomfort and reduce fever.

Hygiene Practices: Keeping the affected area clean and dry is important to prevent the spread of infection. Washing hands frequently and avoiding sharing personal items can also help prevent the spread of bacteria.

In severe cases or if complications arise, such as the development of cellulitis or the spread of infection to other parts of the body, hospitalization and intravenous antibiotics may be necessary.

❖ ❖ ❖ ❖

CELLULITIS (सल्लुलिटिस)

Cellulitis in Ayurveda

Cellulitis, known as "अंगमर्मशोथ" in Ayurveda, is a condition characterized by inflammation of the skin and underlying tissues. According to Ayurveda, cellulitis is primarily caused by an imbalance in the body's doshas, particularly Vata and Kapha.

In Ayurvedic philosophy, Vata governs movement and Kapha governs structure. When these doshas become aggravated due to factors like poor digestion, weakened immunity, or toxins in the body, they can manifest as cellulitis.

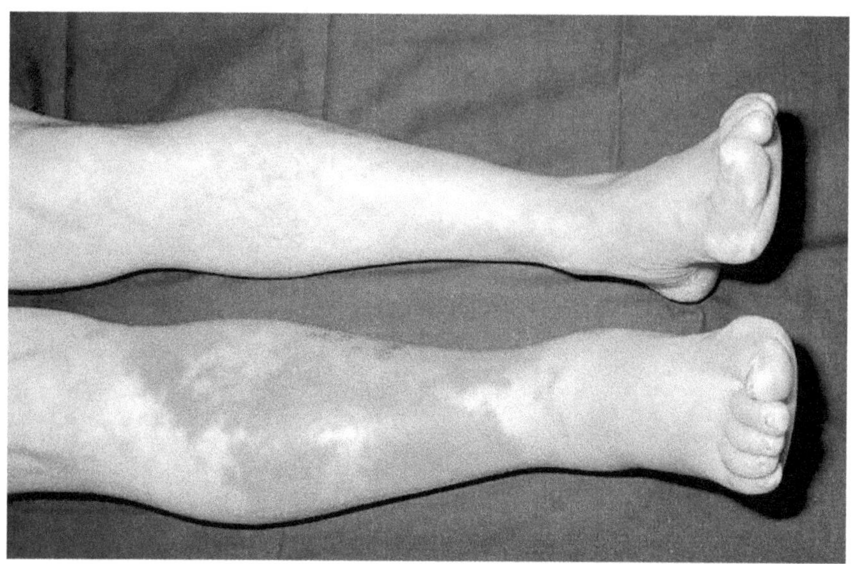

Symptoms of cellulitis according to Ayurveda include redness, swelling, pain, and heat in the affected area. Ayurvedic texts classify cellulitis as a type of **"Vata-Kaphaja Vyadhi"** or disorder caused by the vitiation of both Vata and Kapha doshas.

Ayurvedic treatment for cellulitis focuses on balancing the aggravated doshas and eliminating toxins from the body. This often involves a combination of dietary modifications, herbal remedies, lifestyle changes, and external therapies.

Herbal remedies commonly used in Ayurveda for treating cellulitis include Triphala, Guggulu, Guduchi, Turmeric, and Neem. These herbs possess anti-inflammatory, antimicrobial, and detoxifying properties, which help in reducing inflammation, fighting infections, and promoting healing.

Dietary recommendations for managing cellulitis in Ayurveda emphasize consuming warm, easily digestible foods and avoiding cold, heavy, and processed foods. Drinking warm water infused with ginger or cumin seeds can help improve digestion and detoxification.

Lifestyle modifications such as practicing regular exercise, maintaining proper hygiene, getting adequate rest, and managing stress are also essential for managing cellulitis according to Ayurveda.

External therapies such as Ayurvedic massage (Abhyanga) with medicated oils like Mahanarayan oil or Ksheerabala oil, along with herbal poultices (Upanaha) and fomentation (Swedana), can help alleviate pain, reduce swelling, and promote tissue healing.

Cellulitis in Modern Medicine

Cellulitis in modern medicine is a bacterial skin infection that affects the deeper layers of the skin and the underlying tissue. It is typically caused by bacteria entering the skin through a cut, scrape, or other break in the skin's barrier. The most common bacteria responsible for cellulitis are Streptococcus and Staphylococcus aureus.

Symptoms of Cellulitis Include redness, swelling, warmth, and tenderness in the affected area. As the infection progresses, it can cause fever, chills, and swollen lymph nodes.

Treatment for Cellulitis in modern medicine usually involves antibiotics to eradicate the bacterial infection. Depending on the severity of the infection, oral antibiotics may be sufficient, or intravenous antibiotics may be necessary for more serious cases. Pain relievers may also be prescribed to alleviate discomfort.

In addition to antibiotics, supportive measures such as elevating the affected limb, applying warm compresses to the area, and keeping the area clean and dry are recommended to help reduce swelling and promote healing.

In some cases, cellulitis can lead to complications such as abscess formation, tissue damage, or the spread of infection to the bloodstream (sepsis). Prompt medical attention is essential to prevent complications and ensure proper treatment.

Preventive measures for cellulitis include maintaining good hygiene, promptly treating any cuts or wounds, avoiding tight-fitting clothing that can cause chafing, and managing underlying conditions such as diabetes or immune system disorders that may increase the risk of infection.

Overall, cellulitis in modern medicine is treated with a combination of antibiotics and supportive care aimed at eliminating the bacterial infection and promoting healing of the affected skin and tissue.

❖ ❖ ❖ ❖

CHEILITIS (ओष्ठपाक)

Cheilitis According to Ayurveda

According to Ayurveda, cheilitis is typically associated with an imbalance in the body's doshas – Vata, Pitta, and Kapha. Each dosha governs different physiological functions, and when they are imbalanced, it can lead to various health issues, including cheilitis.

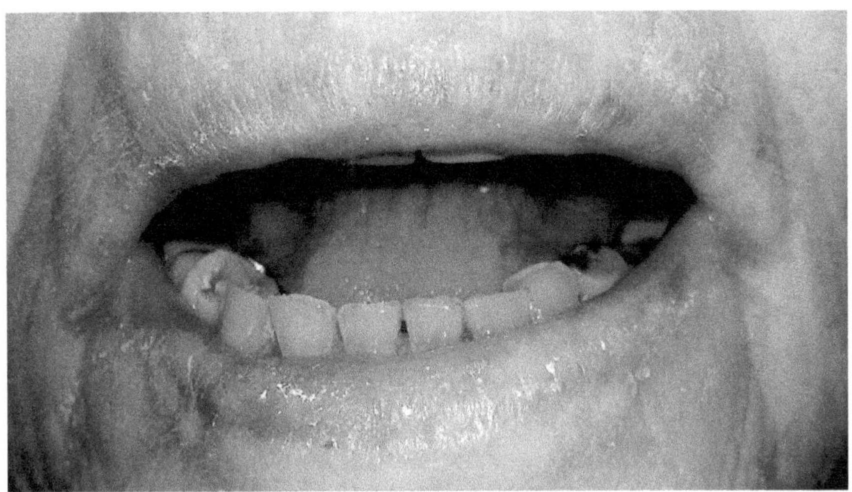

In Ayurveda, the lips are considered a site where several body systems converge, including the digestive system, circulatory system, and nervous system. Therefore, imbalances in any of these systems can manifest as lip disorders like cheilitis.

Ayurvedic Diagnosis of Cheilitis:

Vata Imbalance: When there's an excess of Vata dosha, it can lead to dryness, cracking, and flakiness of the lips. This may be exacerbated by factors such as cold weather, dehydration, and excessive intake of dry, light, and cold foods.

Pitta Imbalance: Excessive Pitta dosha can result in inflammation, redness, and burning sensation on the lips. This may be aggravated by spicy, hot, and acidic foods, as well as exposure to excessive sunlight.

Kapha Imbalance: Kapha imbalance can cause swelling, heaviness, and excessive moisture on the lips. This may occur due to poor digestion, congestion in the body, or overconsumption of heavy, oily, and sweet foods.

Ayurvedic Treatment Approach:

Balancing The Doshas: The primary goal of Ayurvedic treatment is to restore the balance of the doshas. This can be achieved through dietary and lifestyle modifications tailored to each individual's constitution (prakriti) and current imbalances (vikriti).

Herbal Remedies: Various herbs and herbal formulations can be used to address specific doshic imbalances and alleviate symptoms of cheilitis. For example, Aloe vera gel or coconut oil can soothe dry and cracked lips, while herbs like Neem and Manjistha have anti-inflammatory properties that help reduce redness and inflammation.

Dietary Recommendations: Following a diet that pacifies the aggravated doshas is crucial for managing cheilitis. This may involve avoiding foods that are excessively dry, spicy, or oily, and incorporating nourishing and hydrating foods such as fresh fruits, vegetables, whole grains, and healthy fats.

Hydration: Proper hydration is essential for maintaining lip health. Drinking plenty of warm water throughout the day helps to keep the body hydrated and supports the natural moisture balance of the lips.

Stress Management: Stress can exacerbate imbalances in the doshas, so incorporating stress-reducing practices such as meditation, yoga, and deep breathing exercises can be beneficial for managing cheilitis.

Oil Pulling: This ancient Ayurvedic practice involves swishing oil (such as sesame or coconut oil) in the mouth to remove toxins and improve oral hygiene. Oil pulling can help reduce inflammation and promote healing of the lips.

Cheilitis in Modern Science

Cheilitis, as understood in modern science, refers to inflammation of the lips. It can manifest in various forms, including dryness, cracking, redness, swelling, and sometimes blistering or ulcers. Modern medicine recognizes several types of cheilitis, each with its own causes and treatment approaches:

Angular Cheilitis: This type of cheilitis affects the corners of the mouth and is often caused by fungal or bacterial infections, nutritional deficiencies (such as deficiencies in iron, zinc, or B vitamins), or excessive moisture from saliva. Treatment typically involves addressing the underlying cause, such as antifungal or antibacterial medications, topical creams, and dietary supplements.

Actinic Cheilitis: Also known as "solar cheilitis," this condition is caused by long-term sun exposure and primarily affects the lower lip. It can lead to dryness, cracking, and precancerous changes in the lip tissue. Treatment may involve protecting the lips from sun exposure with sunscreen or lip balms containing SPF, as well as regular monitoring by a dermatologist.

Allergic Contact Cheilitis: This form of cheilitis occurs when the lips come into contact with an allergen, such as certain cosmetics, lip balms, toothpaste ingredients, or metals (e.g., nickel). Symptoms include redness, swelling, itching, and sometimes blistering. Treatment involves identifying and avoiding the triggering allergen and may include topical corticosteroids to reduce inflammation.

Cheilitis Granulomatosa: This rare type of cheilitis is characterized by painless, non-tender swelling of the lips and is often associated with conditions like Crohn's disease or sarcoidosis. Treatment may involve oral corticosteroids, immunosuppressive medications, or surgical intervention in severe cases.

Exfoliative Cheilitis: In this condition, the lips become excessively dry and flaky, often with a thickened, whitish layer of skin that can be peeled off. The exact cause is unknown, but factors such as chronic lip licking, infections, or psychological factors may contribute. Treatment may include topical moisturizers, antifungal or antibacterial medications if infection is present, and behavioral therapy to address underlying habits.

Cheilitis Glandularis: This type of cheilitis involves enlargement of the minor salivary glands in the lips, leading to swelling, redness, and sometimes ulceration. It may be associated with conditions like Sjögren's syndrome or chronic sun exposure. Treatment depends on the underlying cause and may involve topical or systemic medications to reduce inflammation.

❖ ❖ ❖ ❖

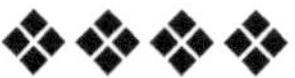

CHICKEN POX (लघुमसुरिका)

Chicken Pox According to Ayurveda

Chickenpox, known as "laghu masurika" in Ayurveda, is a contagious viral infection caused by the varicella-zoster virus. In Ayurveda, it is considered a Pitta-Kapha predominant condition, characterized by symptoms such as fever, rash, and itching. Ayurveda offers a holistic approach to managing chickenpox, focusing on balancing the body's doshas (energies) and strengthening the immune system.

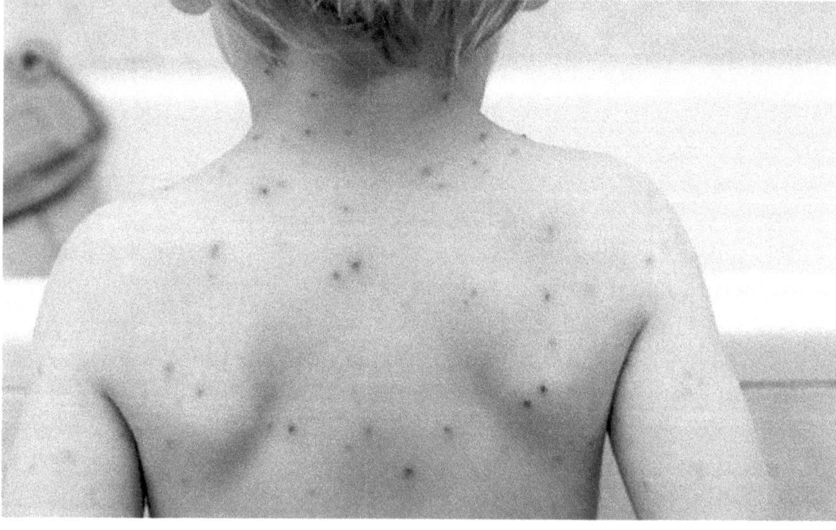

Introduction: Chickenpox, an infectious disease primarily affecting children, manifests with characteristic symptoms like fever, rash, and itching. In Ayurveda, it is classified under "Jwara" (fever) and "Kushta" (skin diseases) and is believed to be caused by an imbalance in the body's doshas, primarily Pitta and Kapha.

Etiology (Nidana: According to Ayurveda, the primary cause of chickenpox is the aggravation of Pitta and Kapha doshas. Factors such as improper diet, lifestyle, seasonal changes, and exposure to pathogens contribute to this imbalance. Contaminated air and contact with infected individuals are also considered contributing factors.

Pathogenesis (Samprapti): When Pitta and Kapha doshas become imbalanced, they accumulate in the skin and blood tissues, leading to the manifestation of chickenpox symptoms. The varicella-zoster virus further exacerbates this imbalance, causing inflammation and eruption of rashes on the skin.

Symptoms (Lakshana): Chickenpox typically begins with symptoms resembling a common cold, such as fever, headache, and malaise. Within a day or two, characteristic red spots or blisters appear on the skin, accompanied by intense itching. These blisters eventually turn into scabs and crusts as the infection progresses.

Ayurvedic Management: Ayurveda emphasizes a comprehensive approach to managing chickenpox, focusing on alleviating symptoms, strengthening the immune system, and restoring dosha balance. The following are key aspects of Ayurvedic management:

Dietary Modifications (Ahara): During chickenpox, it is essential to consume easily digestible, light, and nourishing foods. This includes soups, steamed vegetables, fresh fruits, herbal teas, and warm spices like ginger and turmeric. Avoiding spicy, oily, and heavy foods is crucial to prevent aggravation of Pitta and Kapha.

Herbal Remedies (Aushadha): Ayurvedic herbs such as neem (Azadirachta indica), tulsi (Holy basil), guduchi (Tinospora cordifolia), and manjistha (Rubia cordifolia) are beneficial in managing chickenpox. These herbs possess anti-inflammatory, antiviral, and immune-stimulating properties, aiding in symptom relief and faster recovery.

External Applications (Abhyanga): External application of cooling and soothing herbal oils like coconut oil infused with neem or sandalwood can help alleviate itching and promote healing of the skin lesions. Bathing with neem or oatmeal-infused water can also provide relief from itching and discomfort.

Ayurvedic Preparations (Aushadha Yoga): Ayurvedic formulations such as Gandhak Rasayana, Mahamanjisthadi Kashayam, and Sudarshan Churna may be prescribed by an Ayurvedic practitioner to boost immunity, reduce fever, and promote skin healing.

Lifestyle Modifications (Vihara): Adequate rest and hydration are essential during the recovery period. Avoiding scratching the blisters to prevent secondary infections and scarring is crucial. Maintaining personal hygiene and avoiding close contact with others until the contagious period ends are also important preventive measures.

Chicken Pox in Modern Medicine

Chickenpox, a highly contagious viral infection caused by the varicella-zoster virus (VZV), is widely understood and managed in modern medicine.

Introduction: Chickenpox, also known as varicella, is a common childhood illness characterized by fever and a blister-like rash. It is caused by the varicella-zoster virus, a member of the herpesvirus family. Although chickenpox is usually a mild and self-limiting disease, it can lead to complications, especially in high-risk individuals such as pregnant women, newborns, and individuals with weakened immune systems.

Epidemiology and Transmission: Chickenpox is highly contagious and spreads through respiratory droplets or direct contact with the fluid from the blisters of an infected person. It predominantly affects children, but adults can also contract the virus if they have not been previously infected or vaccinated against it. The incidence of chickenpox has decreased significantly since the introduction of the varicella vaccine.

Clinical Presentation: The typical clinical presentation of chickenpox includes a prodromal phase characterized by fever, malaise, headache, and loss of appetite. Within 24-48 hours, a rash appears, initially consisting of red papules that evolve into fluid-filled vesicles and then crust over. The rash typically starts on the face, scalp, and trunk, spreading to the extremities. It is accompanied by intense itching, which can lead to scratching and potential bacterial superinfection.

Diagnosis: Diagnosing chickenpox is primarily based on clinical presentation, including the characteristic rash and associated symptoms. Laboratory tests such as viral culture or polymerase chain reaction (PCR) may be performed in certain cases, especially when the diagnosis is uncertain or complications are suspected.

Management: The management of chickenpox in modern medicine focuses on alleviating symptoms, preventing complications, and reducing transmission. Treatment may include:

Symptomatic Relief: Over-the-counter medications such as acetaminophen or ibuprofen can be used to reduce fever and alleviate discomfort. Calamine lotion or antihistamines may help relieve itching.

Antiviral Therapy: Antiviral medications such as acyclovir may be prescribed, especially in high-risk individuals or cases with complications. Early initiation of antiviral therapy can shorten the duration of symptoms and reduce the risk of complications.

Preventive Measures: Isolation of infected individuals, good hand hygiene, and avoiding contact with high-risk individuals are crucial to prevent the spread of chickenpox. Vaccination with the varicella vaccine is highly effective in preventing chickenpox and its complications.

Complications Management: Complications of chickenpox, such as bacterial skin infections, pneumonia, encephalitis, or secondary varicella-zoster virus infections (e.g., shingles), may require specific treatments tailored to the individual's condition.

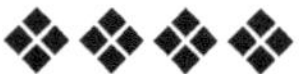

CORN (अट्टन) AND CALLUS

Corn and Callus in Ayurveda

In Ayurveda, corns and calluses are understood within the context of body imbalances and dosha disturbances. These conditions are believed to result from the accumulation of excess Vata and Kapha doshas in the affected areas, leading to the hardening and thickening of the skin.

Corns and calluses are commonly associated with excessive pressure or friction on the skin, often due to ill-fitting footwear or repetitive movements. According to Ayurveda, this pressure disrupts the flow of energy (prana) in the affected areas, causing localized imbalance and subsequent thickening of the skin.

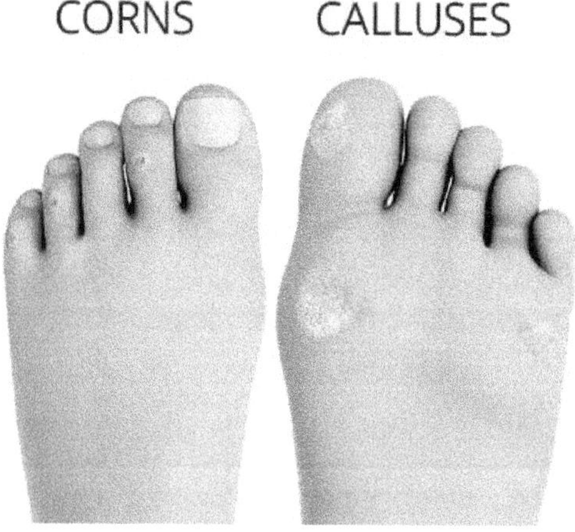

Ayurvedic treatment for corns and calluses typically involves a holistic approach aimed at restoring balance to the affected doshas and promoting overall well-being. Here are some common Ayurvedic remedies and practices for managing corns and calluses:

Dietary Adjustments: Ayurveda emphasizes the importance of diet in maintaining dosha balance. Individuals with corns and calluses are advised to avoid foods that aggravate Vata and Kapha doshas, such as excessively dry or oily foods. Instead, they are encouraged to consume warm, nourishing foods that pacify these doshas.

Herbal Remedies: Various herbs and herbal preparations are used in Ayurveda to alleviate the symptoms of corns and calluses. Some commonly recommended herbs include neem, turmeric, and triphala. These herbs are believed to possess anti-inflammatory and antimicrobial properties, which can help reduce swelling and prevent infection in the affected areas.

External Treatments: Ayurvedic therapies such as oil massage (abhyanga) and herbal poultices (lepa) are often used to soften the hardened skin and promote its natural shedding. Oils such as castor oil or sesame oil are commonly used for massage, as they help nourish the skin and improve circulation to the affected area.

Lifestyle Modifications: Making changes to daily habits and lifestyle can also support the healing process. This may include wearing properly fitted footwear, avoiding repetitive activities that exacerbate the condition, and practicing stress-reducing techniques such as yoga and meditation.

Panchakarma: In severe cases or chronic conditions, Ayurvedic practitioners may recommend Panchakarma therapies to detoxify the body and rebalance the doshas. Panchakarma treatments such as basti (enema therapy) and virechana (therapeutic purgation) can help eliminate accumulated toxins and restore harmony to the body.

Corn and Callus in Modern Science

In modern science, corns and calluses are primarily understood as areas of thickened skin that develop in response to repeated friction or pressure. They are commonly caused by wearing ill-fitting shoes, engaging in repetitive activities, or walking barefoot on hard surfaces.

Corns typically develop on the toes or other bony areas of the foot and have a central core, which may press on nerve endings, causing pain. Calluses, on the other hand, are broader areas of thickened skin that usually form on the soles of the feet or the palms of the hands.

The primary goal of modern medical treatment for corns and calluses is to alleviate discomfort and reduce the risk of complications, such as infection or ulceration. Some common approaches include:

Footwear Modifications: Wearing properly fitted shoes with adequate cushioning and support can help reduce pressure on the feet and prevent the formation of corns and calluses.

Padding and Cushioning: Padding or cushioning devices, such as moleskin or gel inserts, can provide additional protection and reduce friction on areas prone to corns and calluses.

Topical Treatments: Over-the-counter products containing salicylic acid or urea may be used to soften and gradually remove thickened skin. In some cases, a healthcare provider may prescribe stronger topical medications or recommend professional debridement of the affected area.

Orthotic Devices: Custom orthotic devices or shoe inserts may be recommended to redistribute pressure and improve foot biomechanics, thereby reducing the risk of corns and calluses.

Surgical Intervention: In rare cases where conservative measures fail to provide relief, surgical removal of the corn or callus may be considered, particularly if it is causing significant pain or interfering with daily activities.

Preventive measures, such as maintaining good foot hygiene, wearing properly fitting footwear, and avoiding repetitive activities that cause friction or pressure on the skin, are also important in managing corns and calluses.

While modern medical treatments focus primarily on symptom management, they do not necessarily address underlying factors that contribute to the development of corns and calluses.

❖ ❖ ❖ ❖

DANDRUFF (दारुणक)

Dandruff According to Ayurveda

Dandruff, known as "Darunaka" in Ayurveda, is a common scalp disorder characterized by flaking of dead skin cells from the scalp. According to Ayurveda, dandruff is primarily caused by an imbalance in the doshas, specifically the Vata and Kapha doshas.

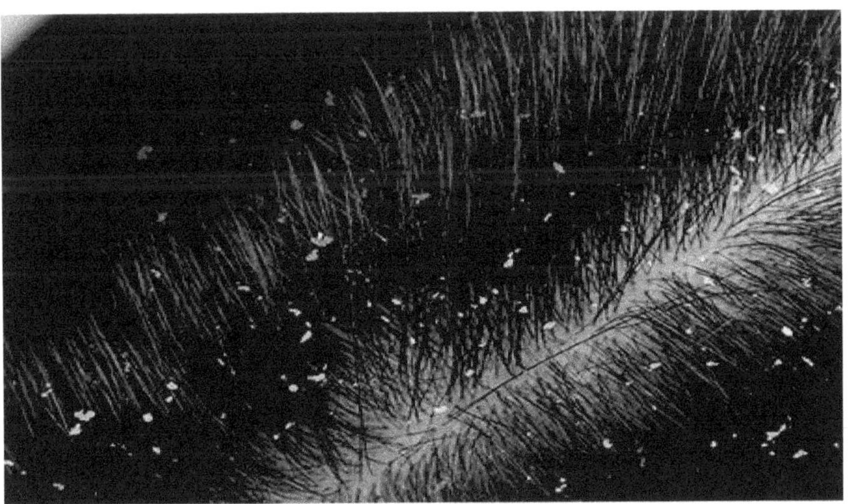

Dosha Imbalance: Ayurveda views dandruff as a result of an imbalance in the doshas, particularly Vata and Kapha. When these doshas are aggravated, they lead to dryness and flakiness of the scalp (Vata imbalance) or excessive oiliness and itching (Kapha imbalance).

Agni (Digestive Fire) Dysfunction: Digestive issues can also contribute to dandruff according to Ayurveda. Poor digestion can lead to the accumulation of toxins in the body, which can manifest as dandruff on the scalp.

Dietary Factors: Ayurveda emphasizes the role of diet in maintaining overall health, including scalp health. Consuming excessive spicy, oily, and fried foods, as well as sugary and fermented foods, can aggravate Pitta dosha and contribute to dandruff.

Lifestyle Factors: Certain lifestyle habits such as irregular sleep patterns, stress, and inadequate hygiene practices can also contribute to dandruff according to Ayurveda.

Herbal Remedies: Ayurveda offers a variety of herbal remedies to treat dandruff. Some commonly used herbs include neem, aloe vera, fenugreek, tulsi (holy basil), and triphala. These herbs possess antimicrobial, anti-inflammatory, and soothing properties that help in alleviating dandruff symptoms.

Oil Massage (Abhyanga): Regular oil massage of the scalp with medicated oils such as coconut oil, sesame oil, or neem oil is recommended in Ayurveda to nourish the scalp, improve circulation, and maintain its health.

Ayurvedic Cleansing (Shiro Abhyanga): Cleansing the scalp with herbal formulations such as shikakai, reetha, and amla can help in removing excess oil, dirt, and dead skin cells, thereby reducing dandruff.

Dietary Recommendations: Ayurveda suggests adopting a Pitta-pacifying diet, which includes cooling and hydrating foods such as fresh fruits, vegetables, whole grains, and plenty of water. Avoiding spicy, oily, and processed foods can help balance Pitta dosha and alleviate dandruff.

Stress Management: Practicing stress-reducing techniques such as yoga, meditation, and pranayama (breathing exercises) can help in managing stress, which is often a contributing factor to dandruff according to Ayurveda.

Dandruff in Modern Medicine

In modern medicine, dandruff is primarily considered a common scalp condition caused by the overgrowth of a fungus called Malassezia, along with factors such as oily skin, hormonal fluctuations, and certain medical conditions. Here's a detailed overview of dandruff from the perspective of modern medicine:

Fungal Overgrowth: Malassezia is a yeast-like fungus found on the scalp of most adults. In individuals prone to dandruff, this fungus can proliferate, leading to an inflammatory response from the immune system and causing flaking of the scalp.

Seborrheic Dermatitis: Dandruff is often associated with seborrheic dermatitis, a common skin condition characterized by red, greasy skin covered with flaky white or yellow scales. Seborrheic dermatitis can affect not only the scalp but also other areas rich in oil glands, such as the face, ears, and chest.

Oily Scalp: Excessive oil (sebum) production by the scalp glands can create an environment conducive to the growth of Malassezia and contribute to the development of dandruff.

Dry Scalp: While dandruff is commonly associated with oily scalp conditions, it can also occur in individuals with dry scalp due to factors such as harsh weather, dehydration, or excessive use of hair products that strip moisture from the scalp.

Hormonal Factors: Hormonal fluctuations, such as those occurring during puberty, pregnancy, or menopause, can influence sebum production and contribute to dandruff.

Medical Conditions: Certain medical conditions, such as psoriasis, eczema, Parkinson's disease, and HIV/AIDS, are associated with an increased risk of developing dandruff or exacerbating existing symptoms.

Stress and Immune Function: Stress and compromised immune function can exacerbate dandruff symptoms by weakening the body's ability to regulate fungal growth and inflammation on the scalp.

Treatment Options: Modern medicine offers various treatment options for dandruff, including over-the-counter medicated shampoos containing active ingredients such as selenium sulfide, zinc pyrithione, ketoconazole, coal tar, or salicylic acid. These ingredients work by reducing fungal growth, controlling oil production, and exfoliating dead skin cells from the scalp.

Lifestyle Modifications: Simple lifestyle modifications, such as maintaining good scalp hygiene, avoiding excessive use of hair products, and managing stress, can also help in managing dandruff effectively.

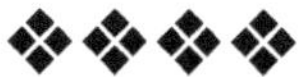

DERMATITIS (क्षुद्र कुष्ठ)

Dermatitis in Ayurveda

Dermatitis, known as "Kshudra Kushtha" in Ayurveda, is a condition where the skin becomes inflamed, red, itchy, and sometimes blistered. According to Ayurveda, derangement of the three doshas – Vata, Pitta, and Kapha – leads to skin disorders like dermatitis.

In Ayurveda, dermatitis is classified into different types based on the predominance of doshas involved:

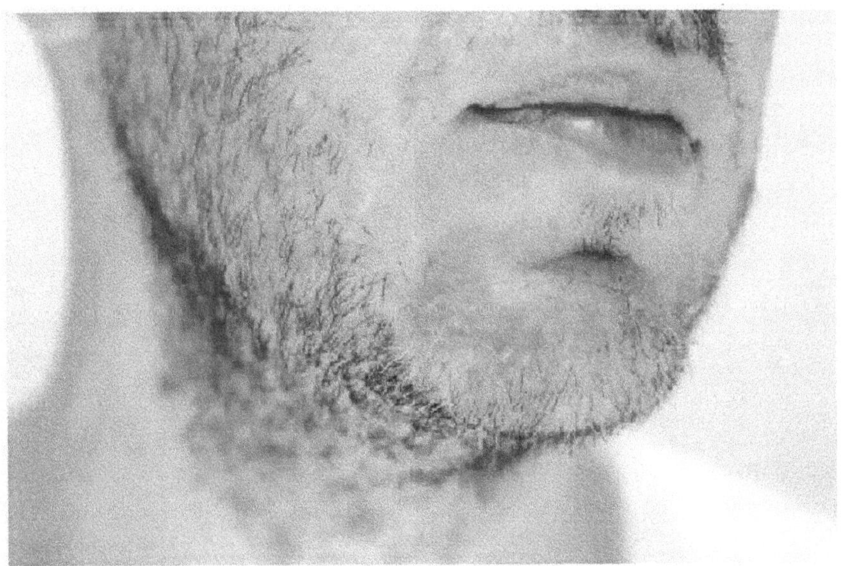

Vataja Kshudra Kushtha: This type of dermatitis is characterized by dry, rough, scaly skin with itching. Vata imbalance leads to decreased oil secretion, causing dryness and flakiness of the skin.

Pittaja Kshudra Kushtha: In this type, there is inflammation, redness, and burning sensation on the skin. Pitta aggravation leads to excess heat in the body, manifesting as inflammatory skin conditions.

Kaphaja Kshudra Kushtha: Kapha imbalance causes excessive oiliness, swelling, and itching in the affected area. There may be oozing of fluid from the lesions.

Sannipataja Kshudra Kushtha: When all three doshas are involved, it leads to a severe and chronic form of dermatitis. The symptoms include a combination of dryness, inflammation, itching, and oozing.

Ayurvedic treatment for dermatitis focuses on restoring the balance of doshas in the body. This includes dietary and lifestyle modifications, herbal remedies, and external therapies such as medicated oils and pastes.

Herbal remedies commonly used in Ayurveda for dermatitis include neem (Azadirachta indica), turmeric (Curcuma longa), aloe vera, manjistha (Rubia cordifolia), and khadir (Acacia catechu). These herbs have anti-inflammatory, anti-microbial, and healing properties that help in relieving symptoms and promoting skin health.

Along with herbal treatments, following a balanced diet, avoiding triggers such as certain foods, harsh chemicals, and environmental allergens, and practicing good skincare habits are essential for managing dermatitis according to Ayurveda. Additionally, stress management techniques such as yoga and meditation can help in reducing flare-ups by calming the mind and balancing the doshas.

Dermatitis in Modern Medicine

In modern medicine, dermatitis refers to a group of inflammatory skin conditions characterized by redness, swelling, itching, and sometimes blistering or oozing. There are several types of dermatitis, including atopic dermatitis (eczema), contact dermatitis (caused by contact with allergens or irritants), seborrheic dermatitis (affecting areas rich in oil glands), and nummular dermatitis (coin-shaped patches of irritated skin).

The exact cause of dermatitis varies depending on the type but can include genetic factors, immune system dysfunction, environmental triggers, and allergies. For example, atopic dermatitis is often associated with a family history of allergic diseases like asthma or hay fever, while contact dermatitis is triggered by direct contact with substances like soaps, detergents, or metals.

Treatment for dermatitis in modern medicine typically involves a combination of approaches, including:

Topical Treatments: These include corticosteroid creams or ointments to reduce inflammation and itching, as well as moisturizers to keep the skin hydrated. In some cases, calcineurin inhibitors or topical immunomodulators may be prescribed.

Oral Medications: For severe cases or those resistant to topical treatments, oral medications such as antihistamines (for itching), antibiotics (for bacterial infections), or immunosuppressants may be prescribed.

Avoidance of Triggers: Identifying and avoiding triggers that exacerbate dermatitis symptoms is crucial. This may involve patch testing to identify allergens in contact dermatitis or keeping a symptom diary to identify triggers in atopic dermatitis.

Phototherapy: In some cases, exposure to certain wavelengths of light (phototherapy) under medical supervision can help improve symptoms of dermatitis, particularly in cases of moderate to severe atopic dermatitis.

Lifestyle Modifications: Practicing good skincare habits, such as using mild cleansers and avoiding harsh soaps or hot water, can help prevent flare-ups. Managing stress and maintaining a healthy diet may also play a role in managing dermatitis symptoms.

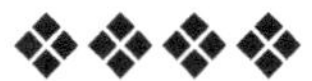

ECZEMA (विचर्चिका)

Eczema in Ayurveda

In Ayurveda, eczema, known as "Vicharchika," is categorized as a "Kshudra Kustha" (minor skin disease) characterized by inflammation, itching, and redness of the skin. Ayurveda views eczema as a manifestation of an imbalance in the body's doshas, particularly Vata and Kapha.

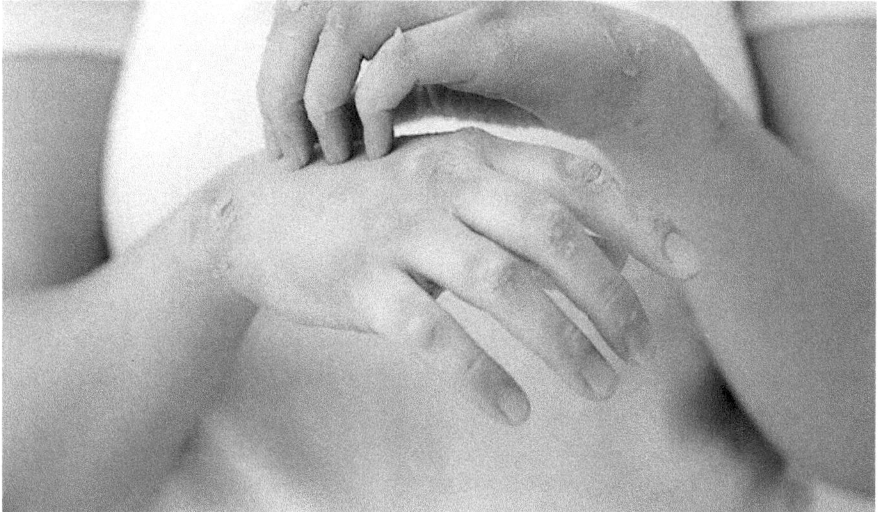

Eczema, or Vicharchika in Ayurveda, is a chronic inflammatory skin condition affecting millions worldwide. According to Ayurveda, eczema is not merely a superficial skin issue but a reflection of deeper imbalances within the body.

Etiology (Nidana): Ayurveda identifies several factors contributing to the development of eczema. These include:

Dosha Imbalance: Imbalance in Vata and Kapha doshas, often aggravated by dietary and lifestyle factors, plays a significant role in triggering eczema.

Improper Diet: Consumption of excessive spicy, oily, and processed foods can aggravate Pitta dosha, contributing to eczema flare-ups.

Toxins (Ama): Accumulation of toxins in the body due to poor digestion and elimination can manifest as skin disorders like eczema.

Stress: Emotional stress and anxiety can weaken the body's immune system, making it more susceptible to eczema.

Environmental Factors: Exposure to harsh weather conditions, allergens, and irritants can exacerbate eczema symptoms.

Pathogenesis (Samprapti): According to Ayurveda, eczema develops through a series of stages involving the doshas, tissues (dhatus), and waste products (malas):

Dosha Imbalance: Aggravation of Vata and Kapha doshas disrupts the normal functioning of the skin, leading to inflammation and itching.

Impaired Digestion: Weak digestion results in the formation of ama (toxins), which circulate in the body and accumulate in the skin, causing inflammation and irritation.

Tissue Involvement: The vitiated doshas affect the deeper tissues (dhatus), particularly the rasa dhatu (plasma) and rakta dhatu (blood), leading to the manifestation of eczema lesions.

Symptom Manifestation: Eczema presents with symptoms such as redness, swelling, vesicles, itching, and dryness, reflecting the underlying doshic imbalance and tissue involvement.

Clinical Features (Rupa): Eczema presents with various clinical features, including:

Dry, Scaly Skin: The affected areas of the skin become dry, scaly, and rough to the touch.

Redness (Rakta): Inflamed patches of skin appear red or pinkish in color due to increased blood circulation.

Itching (Kandu): Intense itching is a hallmark symptom of eczema, leading to scratching and further aggravation of the condition.

Oozing and Crusting: In severe cases, eczema lesions may ooze fluid and form crusts, increasing the risk of infection.

Localized or Generalized: Eczema can affect specific areas of the body or spread to larger areas, depending on individual constitution and severity.

Treatment Approach (Chikitsa): Ayurvedic treatment of eczema aims to balance the doshas, eliminate toxins, nourish the skin, and alleviate symptoms. The treatment modalities include:

Dietary Modification: Emphasizing a diet that pacifies aggravated doshas, including fresh fruits, vegetables, whole grains, and herbal teas. Avoiding spicy, oily, and processed foods is crucial.

Detoxification (Panchakarma): Panchakarma therapies such as Vamana (therapeutic vomiting), Virechana (purgation), and Basti (medicated enema) are employed to eliminate ama and restore doshic balance.

Herbal Remedies: Herbal formulations containing neem, turmeric, aloe vera, and manjistha are used internally and topically to reduce inflammation, itching, and dryness.

Lifestyle Modification: Stress management techniques such as yoga, meditation, and deep breathing exercises help alleviate emotional stress and promote overall well-being.

External Therapies: Application of medicated oils, herbal pastes, and soothing creams helps moisturize the skin, reduce itching, and promote healing of eczema lesions.

Avoidance of Triggers: Identifying and avoiding triggers such as allergens, harsh chemicals, and environmental pollutants is essential to prevent eczema flare-ups.

Conclusion: In conclusion, eczema, or Vicharchika, is a complex skin disorder with multifactorial etiology according to Ayurveda. By addressing the underlying doshic imbalances, promoting detoxification, and adopting a holistic approach to treatment, Ayurveda offers effective management strategies for eczema, restoring skin health and overall well-being.

In modern science, eczema is a chronic inflammatory skin condition characterized by redness, itching, and the formation of dry, scaly patches on the skin. It is often referred to as atopic dermatitis, and its exact cause is not fully understood. However, a combination of genetic, environmental, and immune system factors is believed to play a role in its development.

Etiology:

Genetic Factors: Individuals with a family history of eczema, asthma, or allergies are more likely to develop the condition, suggesting a genetic predisposition.

Immune System Dysfunction: Eczema is associated with immune system dysregulation, leading to an abnormal inflammatory response in the skin.

Environmental Triggers: Exposure to irritants, allergens, harsh chemicals, and certain fabrics can trigger or exacerbate eczema symptoms.

Skin Barrier Dysfunction: Impairment of the skin's barrier function allows moisture to escape and irritants to penetrate, leading to inflammation and itching.

Pathophysiology:

Skin Inflammation: Eczema is characterized by inflammation of the skin, driven by an overactive immune response involving T cells and cytokines.

Skin Barrier Defects: Defects in the skin barrier allow allergens, irritants, and microbes to penetrate the skin, triggering an inflammatory cascade.

Itch-Scratch Cycle: Itching is a hallmark symptom of eczema, leading to scratching, which further damages the skin barrier and exacerbates inflammation.

Microbial Colonization: Bacterial and fungal colonization of the skin may contribute to the pathogenesis of eczema, leading to secondary infections and worsening of symptoms.

Clinical Features:

Redness and Inflammation: Affected areas of the skin appear red, inflamed, and may develop small bumps or blisters.

Itching: Intense itching is a prominent symptom of eczema, often leading to scratching and exacerbation of the condition.

Dry, Scaly Skin: Eczema patches are typically dry, scaly, and may crack or weep fluid in severe cases.

Distribution: Eczema can affect any part of the body but commonly occurs on the face, hands, elbows, knees, and behind the knees.

Treatment:

Topical Corticosteroids: Corticosteroid creams or ointments are often prescribed to reduce inflammation and itching during eczema flare-ups.

Moisturizers: Regular use of moisturizers helps hydrate the skin and restore the skin barrier function, reducing dryness and itching.

Topical Calcineurin Inhibitors: These medications inhibit the immune response in the skin, helping to reduce inflammation and itching.

Antihistamines: Oral antihistamines may be prescribed to relieve itching and improve sleep quality in patients with eczema.

Avoidance of Triggers: Identifying and avoiding triggers such as irritants, allergens, and harsh skincare products is essential to prevent eczema flare-ups.

Lifestyle Modifications: Keeping the skin well-hydrated, avoiding hot showers, and wearing soft, breathable fabrics can help manage eczema symptoms.

❖ ❖ ❖ ❖

ERYSIPELAS (विसर्प)

Erysipelas According to Ayurveda

Erysipelas, known as "Visarpa" in Ayurveda, is a condition characterized by inflammation of the skin and underlying connective tissue, typically caused by Streptococcus bacteria. In Ayurveda, it is classified under the category of "Kushtha," which refers to various skin diseases.

According to Ayurvedic principles, Visarpa is caused due to an imbalance in the body's doshas, primarily Pitta and Kapha. When these doshas become aggravated, they impair the digestive fire (Agni), leading to the accumulation of toxins (Ama) in the body. This accumulation weakens the immune system and creates a favorable environment for the growth of harmful bacteria, leading to conditions like Visarpa.

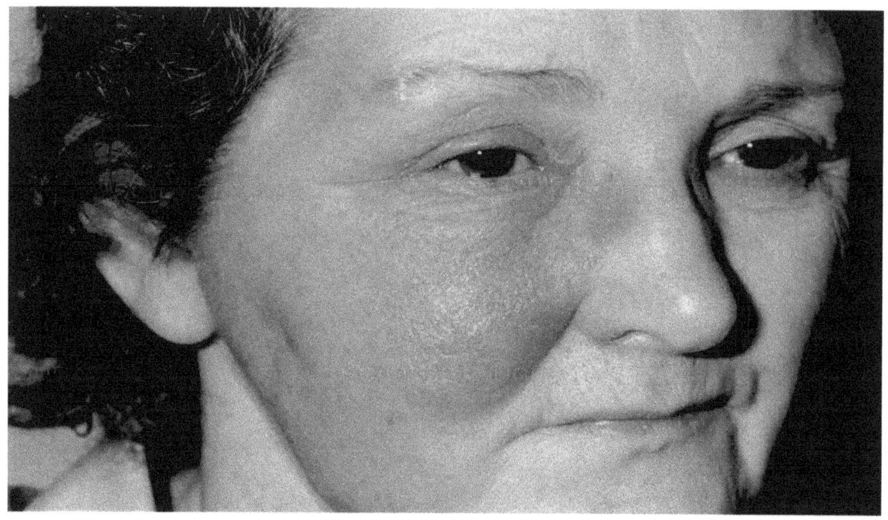

The symptoms of Visarpa, as described in Ayurvedic texts, include redness, swelling, severe pain, and heat in the affected area. There may also be fever, chills, and general malaise. These symptoms are indicative of an imbalance in Pitta and Kapha doshas.

Ayurvedic treatment for Visarpa focuses on restoring the balance of doshas and eliminating toxins from the body. The approach includes:

Panchakarma Therapy: This is a detoxification therapy aimed at eliminating toxins from the body. It includes procedures like Vamana (therapeutic vomiting), Virechana (purgation), and Rakta Mokshana (bloodletting) to remove excess Pitta and Kapha from the body.

Herbal Remedies: Ayurveda prescribes various herbs with anti-inflammatory, antibacterial, and detoxifying properties to treat Visarpa. These may include Neem (Azadirachta indica), Turmeric (Curcuma longa), Giloy (Tinospora cordifolia), Manjistha (Rubia cordifolia), and Guduchi (Tinospora cordifolia).

Dietary Modifications: Diet plays a crucial role in managing Visarpa. Ayurveda recommends consuming cooling and Pitta-pacifying foods such as fresh fruits, vegetables, whole grains, and herbal teas. Spicy, oily, and fried foods should be avoided as they can aggravate Pitta.

Lifestyle Changes: Stress management techniques, regular exercise, and adequate rest are essential for maintaining overall health and supporting the body's natural healing process.

External Therapies: Local applications of herbal pastes, oils, and poultices may help reduce inflammation, relieve pain, and promote healing of the affected skin.

Preventive Measures: Practicing good hygiene, avoiding contact with infected individuals, and keeping the skin clean and moisturized can help prevent the recurrence of Visarpa.

In conclusion, Ayurveda offers a holistic approach to the management of Visarpa, focusing on restoring the balance of doshas, eliminating toxins, and promoting overall health and well-being.

Erysipelas in Modern Medicine

Erysipelas, known as "Visarpa" in Ayurveda, is a bacterial infection of the skin and underlying tissues. In modern medicine, it is primarily caused by group A Streptococcus bacterium, although other types of bacteria can also be responsible. Erysipelas typically affects the face, legs, arms, or other areas of the body, causing redness, swelling, warmth, and pain.

The infection usually starts with a break in the skin, such as a cut, scrape, or insect bite, which allows the bacteria to enter the body and multiply. Factors that increase the risk of developing erysipelas include compromised immune function, chronic skin conditions, obesity, and lymphedema.

The diagnosis of erysipelas is based on clinical examination, including the characteristic appearance of the affected area and the presence of symptoms such as fever and chills. In some cases, a sample of the affected skin may be taken for laboratory testing to confirm the presence of bacteria.

Treatment for erysipelas typically involves antibiotics to eradicate the infection. Depending on the severity of the infection, antibiotics may be prescribed orally or administered intravenously. Pain relievers and anti-inflammatory medications may also be recommended to alleviate symptoms such as pain and swelling.

In addition to antibiotic therapy, supportive measures such as rest, elevation of the affected limb, and proper wound care are important for promoting healing and preventing complications. In severe cases or in individuals with underlying health conditions, hospitalization may be necessary for close monitoring and intravenous antibiotics.

❖ ❖ ❖ ❖

FRECKLES (तिल)

Freckles in Ayurveda

In Ayurveda, freckles, or "तिल" are considered a manifestation of an imbalance, particularly in Pitta dosha, which governs metabolism and digestion, as well as skin health.

Freckles are believed to arise due to an excess of Pitta dosha, particularly when it becomes aggravated by factors such as exposure to excessive sunlight, consumption of spicy and oily foods, stress, and hormonal fluctuations.

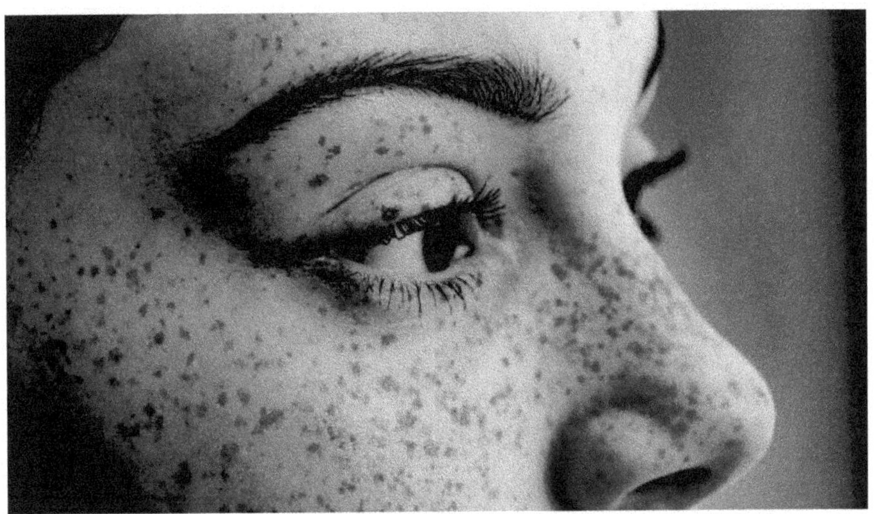

Understanding Pitta Dosha: Pitta is composed of fire and water elements and governs digestion, metabolism, and transformation in the body. When Pitta becomes imbalanced, it can manifest as skin conditions like freckles, acne, and inflammation.

Dietary Recommendations: Ayurveda emphasizes dietary adjustments to pacify aggravated Pitta. This involves favoring cooling, hydrating foods such as fresh fruits and vegetables, whole grains, and herbal teas. Foods that are spicy, oily, and acidic should be minimized, as they can exacerbate Pitta imbalance.

Herbal Remedies: Ayurvedic herbs like Neem, Manjistha, and Aloe Vera are renowned for their Pitta-pacifying and skin-healing properties. These herbs can be consumed internally as supplements or applied topically in the form of pastes or creams to help reduce freckles and promote clear skin.

Lifestyle Modifications: Avoiding excessive sun exposure, particularly during peak hours, is crucial in managing freckles. Wearing protective clothing, using natural sunscreen, and seeking shade when outdoors can help prevent further pigmentation. Additionally, stress management techniques such as yoga, meditation, and breathing exercises can support overall balance and skin health.

Ayurvedic Treatments: Ayurvedic therapies such as Panchakarma, which includes detoxification procedures like Virechana (therapeutic purgation) and Raktamokshana (bloodletting), may be recommended in severe cases of Pitta imbalance and skin disorders like freckles.

Holistic Approach: Ayurveda emphasizes a holistic approach to health, recognizing the interconnectedness of the mind, body, and spirit. Therefore, alongside dietary and lifestyle adjustments, addressing underlying emotional imbalances and promoting mental well-being through practices like mindfulness and self-care is essential in managing conditions like freckles.

Freckles in Modern Medicine

In modern medicine, freckles, or "तिल" are referred to as "ephelides" and are considered harmless pigmented spots on the skin. They are commonly observed in individuals with fair skin and tend to darken with sun exposure. Here's a detailed overview of freckles from a modern medical perspective:

Cause: Freckles are primarily caused by an increase in the production of melanin, the pigment responsible for skin color. Sun exposure stimulates the production of melanin, leading to the development of freckles, especially in areas of the skin that are frequently exposed to sunlight.

Genetic Factors: Genetics play a significant role in the development of freckles. Individuals with fair skin, red or blonde hair, and light-colored eyes are more prone to developing freckles compared to those with darker skin tones.

Sun Exposure: Ultraviolet (UV) radiation from sunlight is a major contributing factor to the formation of freckles. Sun exposure stimulates melanocytes, the cells that produce melanin, to increase melanin production in response to protect the skin from further damage.

Prevention: Prevention of freckles primarily involves sun protection measures, such as wearing sunscreen with a high SPF, seeking shade during peak sunlight hours, wearing protective clothing, and using wide-brimmed hats and sunglasses. These measures help minimize sun-induced skin damage and reduce the risk of freckle formation.

Treatment: While freckles themselves are harmless, some individuals may choose to reduce their appearance for cosmetic reasons. Treatment options may include topical creams or serums containing ingredients like hydroquinone, retinoids, or vitamin C, which can help lighten pigmented spots over time. Additionally, procedures such as laser therapy, chemical peels, or cryotherapy may be used to target and remove freckles, although multiple sessions may be required for optimal results.

Monitoring: It's important to monitor freckles for any changes in size, shape, or color, as these could be signs of skin cancer, particularly melanoma. Regular skin examinations by a dermatologist are recommended, especially for individuals with a history of excessive sun exposure or a family history of skin cancer.

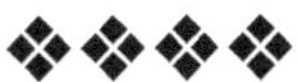

FOLLICULITIS (रोमकूपशोथ)

Folliculitis According to Ayurveda

Folliculitis is a common skin condition characterized by inflammation of the hair follicles. According to Ayurveda, it can be understood through the lens of doshas (Vata, Pitta, and Kapha), dhatus (tissues), and malas (waste products).

Ayurveda views folliculitis as primarily a Pitta disorder, with an imbalance in the fire element. Pitta governs digestion, metabolism, and heat in the body. When Pitta becomes aggravated, it can lead to inflammation and heat-related conditions like folliculitis.

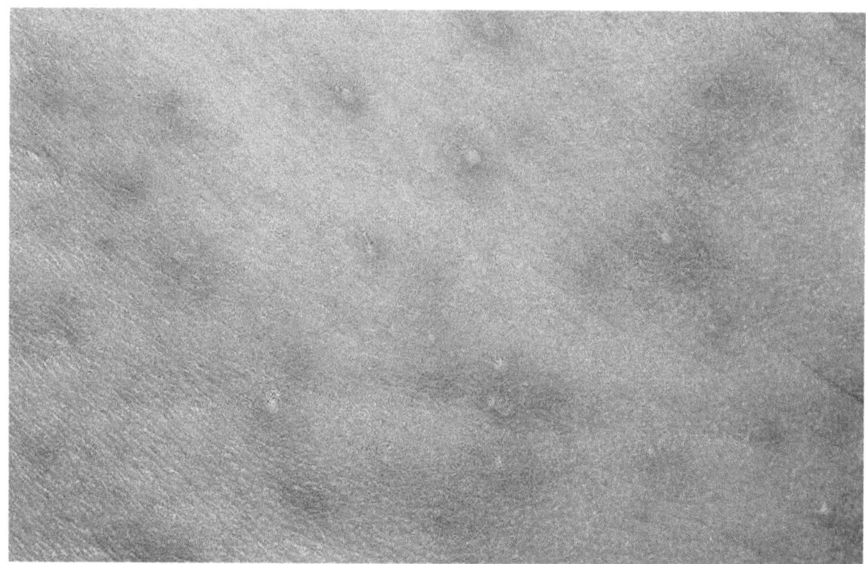

From an Ayurvedic perspective, several factors can contribute to the aggravation of Pitta and the onset of folliculitis:

Dietary Factors: Consuming excessive spicy, oily, and acidic foods can aggravate Pitta dosha. Foods like fried foods, caffeine, alcohol, and acidic fruits may exacerbate inflammation in the body, including the skin.

Poor Digestion: Weak digestion can lead to the accumulation of toxins (ama) in the body, which can further aggravate Pitta. Eating incompatible food combinations or eating in a hurried or stressed state can impair digestion.

Excessive Heat and Sweat: Exposure to excessive heat and sweating can aggravate Pitta and contribute to the inflammation of hair follicles. This may occur due to environmental factors or excessive physical activity.

Stress: Emotional stress and tension can also disturb the balance of Pitta in the body, leading to various skin conditions, including folliculitis.

Treatment

Ayurvedic treatment for folliculitis aims to balance Pitta dosha and alleviate inflammation in the affected area. This may involve dietary modifications, lifestyle changes, herbal remedies, and external therapies. Here are some Ayurvedic approaches to managing folliculitis:

Dietary Recommendations: Emphasize cooling, hydrating foods that pacify Pitta dosha. This includes sweet, bitter, and astringent tastes. Avoid hot, spicy, and oily foods. Drinking plenty of water and consuming foods with high water content, such as cucumber and melons, can help maintain hydration and cool the body.

Herbal Remedies: Ayurvedic herbs like neem, turmeric, aloe vera, and sandalwood have cooling and anti-inflammatory properties that can help soothe inflammation and reduce Pitta in the body. These herbs can be taken internally or applied topically as pastes or oils.

Detoxification: Detoxifying the body through practices like Panchakarma (Ayurvedic detoxification therapies) can help remove ama and balance Pitta dosha. Panchakarma treatments may include oil massages (Abhyanga), steam therapy (Swedana), and herbal enemas (Basti).

Stress Management: Practices like yoga, meditation, and pranayama (breath control) can help reduce stress and promote relaxation, thereby balancing Pitta dosha.

External Care: Topical applications of cooling herbal pastes or oils can help soothe inflammation and promote healing of the affected hair follicles. Gentle exfoliation with natural scrubs can also help remove dead skin cells and prevent further blockage of the follicles.

Folliculitis in Modern Medicine

Folliculitis is a common skin condition in modern medicine characterized by inflammation of the hair follicles. It can occur anywhere on the body where hair follicles are present, leading to symptoms such as redness, itching, and small, pus-filled bumps. The condition can be acute or chronic and may result from bacterial, fungal, or viral infections, as well as other factors.

Causes:

Bacterial Folliculitis: Most cases of folliculitis are caused by bacterial infections, commonly by Staphylococcus aureus. These bacteria can enter the hair follicle through small cuts or breaks in the skin, leading to infection and inflammation. Bacterial folliculitis may be superficial, affecting the upper part of the hair follicle, or deep, involving the deeper layers of the skin.

Fungal Folliculitis: Fungal infections, such as those caused by the yeast Malassezia or dermatophytes, can also lead to folliculitis. These infections are more common in warm and humid environments and may affect areas such as the scalp, groin, and beard area.

Viral Folliculitis: Viral infections, such as herpes simplex virus (HSV) or human papillomavirus (HPV), can occasionally cause folliculitis. These infections may result in clusters of small, painful blisters around the affected hair follicles.

Non-Infectious Folliculitis: Folliculitis can also occur without an infectious cause, due to factors such as physical irritation from shaving, friction from clothing, or exposure to certain chemicals or oils. This type of folliculitis is often referred to as pseudofolliculitis barbae when it occurs in the beard area.

Treatment for folliculitis in modern medicine depends on the underlying cause and severity of the condition. It may include:

Topical Treatments: Mild cases of folliculitis may be treated with topical antibiotics or antifungal medications to reduce inflammation and control infection. Topical corticosteroids may also be prescribed to reduce itching and inflammation.

Oral Medications: In cases of severe or recurrent folliculitis, oral antibiotics or antifungal medications may be prescribed to target the underlying infection. Oral corticosteroids may be used in cases of severe inflammation.

Hygiene Measures: Proper hygiene practices, such as keeping the affected area clean and dry, avoiding tight clothing, and using clean razors, can help prevent folliculitis and reduce its severity.

Lifestyle Modifications: Avoiding activities that exacerbate folliculitis, such as shaving too closely or using harsh chemical products, can help prevent recurrences.

Procedures: In some cases, procedures such as laser hair removal or surgical drainage of abscesses may be necessary for the management of chronic or severe folliculitis.

Overall, modern medicine provides a range of treatment options for folliculitis, tailored to the specific cause and characteristics of the condition. Early diagnosis and appropriate treatment are key to preventing complications and achieving resolution of symptoms.

Premature Greying of Hair According to Ayurveda

In Ayurveda, premature greying of hair, known as "Akala Palitam" or "Palitya," is considered a sign of imbalanced doshas, primarily Pitta and Vata. This condition is attributed to various factors, including dietary habits, lifestyle choices, stress, genetic predisposition, and environmental factors. Ayurveda offers a holistic approach to understanding and treating premature greying by addressing the root cause rather than just the symptoms.

According to Ayurveda, the hair is considered a byproduct of bone tissue (asthi dhatu) and is nourished by the same factors that nourish bones. When there is an imbalance in the doshas, particularly Pitta and Vata, it affects the quality and color of the hair. Excessive Pitta dosha can lead to premature greying due to its heating and inflammatory nature, while Vata imbalance can cause dryness and depletion of melanin, the pigment responsible for hair color.

Diet plays a crucial role in Ayurvedic treatment for premature greying. Foods that aggravate Pitta dosha, such as spicy, oily, and fried foods, should be avoided. Instead, focus on incorporating cooling and nourishing foods like fresh fruits, vegetables, whole grains, and dairy products into your diet. Herbs like Brahmi, Amalaki, Bhringraj, and Aloe Vera are also beneficial for hair health and can help balance the doshas.

Ayurvedic lifestyle practices are essential for preventing and managing premature greying. Maintaining a regular sleep schedule, managing stress through meditation and yoga, and avoiding excessive exposure to heat and sun can help balance Pitta and Vata doshas. Additionally, scalp massages with herbal oils like coconut oil, almond oil, or Brahmi oil can nourish the hair follicles and promote healthy hair growth.

Ayurvedic treatments such as Shirodhara, Nasya, and Shiro Abhyanga (head massage) with herbal oils are recommended for balancing the doshas and rejuvenating the scalp and hair. Panchakarma therapies like Virechana (purification through purgation) and Basti (medicated enema) may also be prescribed by Ayurvedic practitioners to detoxify the body and restore doshic balance.

Premature Greying in Modern Medicine

In modern medicine, premature greying of hair, known as canities, is primarily attributed to genetic factors, environmental influences, and underlying medical conditions. While Ayurveda focuses on holistic approaches and doshic imbalances, modern medicine delves into the physiological and biochemical aspects of premature greying.

Genetics plays a significant role in premature greying, with studies suggesting that variations in genes responsible for melanin production and regulation can predispose individuals to early onset greying. Environmental factors such as exposure to pollutants, ultraviolet (UV) radiation, and oxidative stress can also accelerate the greying process by damaging melanocytes, the cells responsible for producing melanin.

Furthermore, medical conditions such as thyroid disorders, vitiligo, autoimmune diseases, and nutritional deficiencies can contribute to premature greying. For instance, deficiencies in vitamins B12, B6, and D, as well as minerals like iron and copper, can affect melanin synthesis and hair pigmentation.

Oxidative stress, caused by an imbalance between antioxidants and free radicals in the body, is another key factor in premature greying. Free radicals can damage melanocytes and disrupt melanin production, leading to premature greying. Lifestyle factors such as smoking, poor diet, and chronic stress can exacerbate oxidative stress and accelerate the greying process.

Treatment options in modern medicine focus on addressing the underlying cause of premature greying and managing symptoms. This may include lifestyle modifications, such as quitting smoking, improving diet, and managing stress. Additionally, topical treatments containing minoxidil or peptide-based therapies may help stimulate melanocyte activity and promote hair pigmentation.

In cases where medical conditions are contributing to premature greying, treatment may involve addressing the underlying condition through medication or other interventions. For example, thyroid hormone replacement therapy may be prescribed for thyroid disorders, while supplementation with vitamins and minerals may be recommended for nutritional deficiencies.

While modern medicine does not offer a cure for premature greying, various treatments and interventions can help manage the condition and improve the appearance of grey hair. However, more research is needed to fully understand the complex mechanisms underlying premature greying and develop targeted therapies for prevention and treatment.

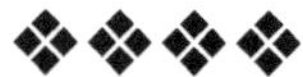

HAIR FALL (खालित्य)

Hair Fall According to Ayurveda

In Ayurveda, hair fall, known as Khalitya, is considered a common problem with multifactorial causes, including imbalances in the doshas (Vata, Pitta, and Kapha), improper diet, stress, poor lifestyle choices, and environmental factors.

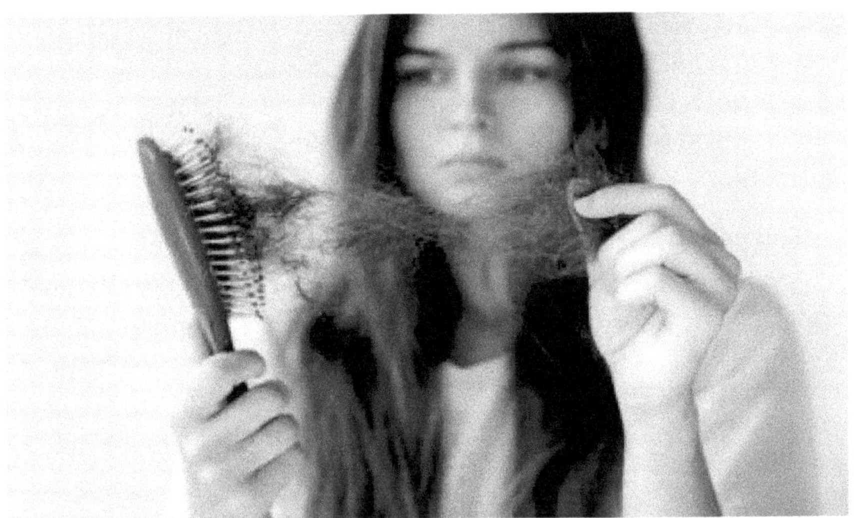

Understanding Khalitya (Hair Fall) In Ayurveda:

Hair fall, or Khalitya, is a prevalent concern affecting both men and women globally. In Ayurveda, it is seen as a manifestation of underlying imbalances within the body. Ayurvedic texts emphasize the importance of maintaining a balance between the three doshas – Vata, Pitta, and Kapha – for overall health and well-being, including the health of the hair and scalp.

Causes of Khalitya According to Ayurveda:

Imbalance of Doshas: Ayurveda attributes hair fall to an imbalance of the doshas. Excessive Vata dosha can lead to dryness and weakness of the hair follicles, resulting in hair fall. Pitta imbalance can cause inflammation of the scalp, leading to conditions like dandruff and premature graying, which contribute to hair loss. Kapha imbalance may lead to excess oiliness and congestion of the scalp, obstructing hair growth.

Dietary Factors: Ayurveda emphasizes the importance of a balanced diet for maintaining healthy hair. Consuming excessive spicy, oily, and processed foods can aggravate Pitta and Kapha doshas, leading to hair fall. Conversely, a diet lacking in essential nutrients such as vitamins, minerals, and proteins can weaken the hair follicles and contribute to hair loss.

Stress and Lifestyle: Chronic stress, inadequate sleep, and unhealthy lifestyle choices can disrupt the body's natural equilibrium, affecting the doshas and weakening the hair follicles. Irregular daily routines, excessive physical and mental exertion, and exposure to environmental toxins can also exacerbate hair fall according to Ayurveda.

Environmental Factors: Exposure to harsh environmental conditions such as pollution, harsh sunlight, and excessive humidity can damage the hair shaft and scalp, leading to hair fall. Additionally, the use of chemical-laden hair products, frequent heat styling, and improper hair care practices can further exacerbate the problem.

Ayurvedic Approach to Managing Khalitya:

Balancing The Doshas: Ayurvedic treatments aim to restore the balance of the doshas through dietary modifications, herbal remedies, lifestyle changes, and therapies such as Panchakarma. Tailored treatment plans are designed based on individual constitution (Prakriti) and imbalances to address the root cause of hair fall.

Herbal Remedies: Ayurveda utilizes a wide range of herbs and herbal formulations to nourish the scalp, strengthen the hair roots, and promote hair growth. Some commonly used herbs for treating Khalitya include Bhringraj (Eclipta alba), Amla (Emblica officinalis), Brahmi (Bacopa monnieri), Neem (Azadirachta indica), and Triphala.

Dietary Recommendations: Ayurveda emphasizes the importance of a balanced and nourishing diet to support hair health. Including foods rich in vitamins, minerals, proteins, and healthy fats such as leafy greens, whole grains, nuts, seeds, and fresh fruits can help strengthen the hair follicles and prevent hair fall.

Stress Management: Stress reduction techniques such as yoga, meditation, and pranayama (breathwork) are integral parts of Ayurvedic management of hair fall. These practices help calm the mind, balance the doshas, and promote overall well-being, which in turn can help reduce hair fall.

Proper Hair Care: Ayurveda advocates for gentle and natural hair care practices to maintain the health of the scalp and hair. This includes regular oil massage (abhyanga) using herbal oils like coconut oil or sesame oil, gentle cleansing with mild herbal shampoos, and avoiding excessive heat styling and chemical treatments.

Hair Fall in Modern Medicine

In modern medicine, hair fall, or alopecia, is approached from a scientific perspective, considering various factors such as genetics, hormonal imbalances, medical conditions, medications, and environmental factors. Here's a detailed essay on hair fall in modern medicine:

Understanding Hair Fall in Modern Medicine:

Hair fall, medically known as alopecia, is a common condition that affects individuals of all ages, genders, and ethnicities worldwide. In modern medicine, hair fall is classified into different types based on its underlying causes, including androgenetic alopecia, alopecia areata, telogen effluvium, and others. Understanding the specific type of alopecia is crucial for determining the most appropriate treatment approach.

Causes Of Hair Fall In Modern Medicine:

Genetics: Androgenetic alopecia, also known as male-pattern or female-pattern baldness, is the most common cause of hair fall and is largely determined by genetics. It involves a combination of genetic predisposition and hormonal factors that lead to progressive hair thinning and eventual baldness.

Hormonal Imbalances: Hormonal imbalances, such as fluctuations in Conditions like polycystic ovary syndrome (PCOS) in women an
d hormonal changes during pregnancy, childbirth, and menopause can also trigger hair loss.

Medical Conditions: Certain medical conditions and diseases can cause hair fall as a secondary symptom. Examples include thyroid disorders (hyperthyroidism or hypothyroidism), autoimmune diseases (e.g., lupus), scalp infections (e.g., ringworm), and nutritional deficiencies (e.g., iron deficiency anemia).

Medications: Some medications, particularly those used in cancer chemotherapy, can cause hair loss as a side effect. Other medications that may contribute to hair fall include certain antidepressants, anticoagulants, beta-blockers, and oral contraceptives.

Stress and Lifestyle Factors: Psychological stress, physical trauma, crash dieting, and extreme weight loss can trigger a condition called telogen effluvium, characterized by excessive shedding of hair. Poor nutrition, smoking, excessive alcohol consumption, and harsh hair care practices can also contribute to hair fall.

Modern Approaches To Managing Hair Fall:

Topical Treatments: Over-the-counter and prescription topical treatments containing minoxidil (Rogaine) are commonly used to promote hair growth and prevent further hair loss in androgenetic alopecia. Other topical medications, such as corticosteroids and anthralin, may be prescribed for specific types of alopecia.

Oral Medications: Finasteride (Propecia) is an oral medication approved for the treatment of androgenetic alopecia in men. It works by blocking the conversion of testosterone into dihydro testosterone, thereby reducing hair loss and promoting hair regrowth. However, it is not recommended for use in women due to potential side effects.

Platelet-Rich Plasma (Prp) Therapy: PRP therapy involves extracting platelets from the patient's blood and injecting them into the scalp to stimulate hair growth. This treatment has gained popularity as a non-surgical option for hair restoration, particularly in cases of androgenetic alopecia and alopecia areata.

Hair Transplantation: Hair transplantation procedures, such as follicular unit transplantation (FUT) and follicular unit extraction (FUE), involve harvesting hair follicles from a donor site (usually the back or sides of the scalp) and transplanting them into the balding areas. This surgical intervention is often considered for individuals with advanced hair loss who seek permanent hair restoration.

Lifestyle Modifications: Adopting a healthy lifestyle, managing stress effectively, maintaining a balanced diet rich in essential nutrients, and avoiding harsh hair care practices can help minimize hair fall and promote overall hair health.

treatment effectiveness and achieving satisfactory outcomes in managing hair fall.

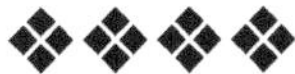

HEEL FISSURE (विपादक)

Heel Fissure According to Ayurveda

Heel fissures, known as "Vipadika" in Ayurveda, are a common condition characterized by cracks or splits in the skin of the heels. In Ayurveda, Vipadika is classified under "Kshudra roga" (minor diseases) and is primarily caused by vitiated Vata dosha, especially when it affects the skin.

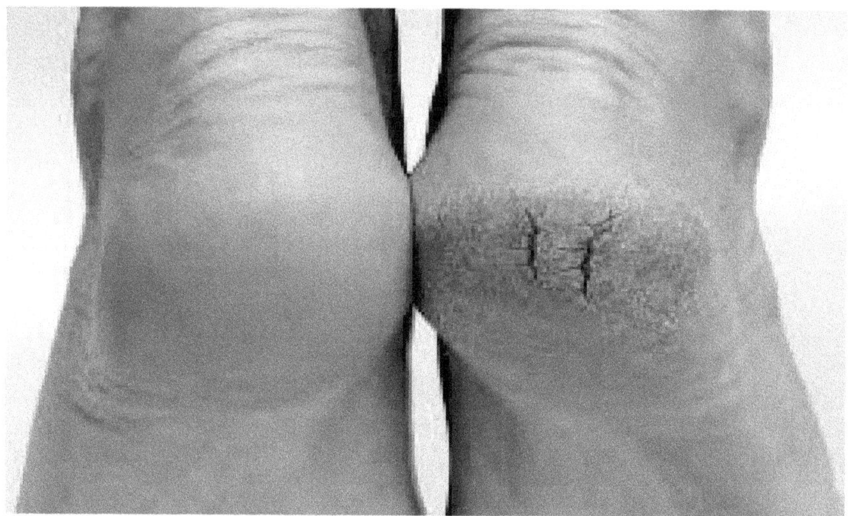

Vata Dosha Imbalance: Vata governs the movement and dryness in the body. When it becomes aggravated, it leads to dryness and roughness in the skin, making it prone to cracks and fissures.

Excessive Walking Or Standing: Overuse of the feet, such as prolonged standing or walking, can lead to pressure on the heels, causing them to crack.

Improper Footwear: Wearing ill-fitting or open-back shoes can contribute to the development of heel fissures by causing friction and pressure on the heels.

Unhealthy Diet: Consumption of dry, rough, and spicy foods can aggravate Vata dosha, further worsening the condition.

Ayurvedic management of Vipadika focuses on pacifying aggravated Vata dosha and promoting the healing of the cracks. Treatment typically includes:

Snehana (Oleation Therapy): External application of medicated oils like Mahanarayana oil or plain coconut oil helps to lubricate the skin, reducing dryness and promoting healing.

Swedana (Fomentation Therapy): This involves applying heat to the affected area, which helps to improve blood circulation and enhance the absorption of oils applied externally.

Lepa (Medicated Paste): Applying medicated pastes made from herbs like Manjistha (Rubia cordifolia) or Yashtimadhu (Glycyrrhiza glabra) helps to soothe the cracked skin and promote healing.

Dietary Modifications: Consuming a diet that pacifies Vata dosha, including warm, nourishing foods and staying hydrated, can help to balance the doshas internally.

Foot Care: Proper foot hygiene, including regular washing and moisturizing of the feet, is essential to prevent further complications and promote healing.

Avoiding Excessive Walking or Standing: Resting the feet and avoiding activities that put excessive pressure on the heels can help to prevent worsening of the condition.

Herbal Supplements: Internal administration of herbs like Guggulu (Commiphora mukul) or Shatavari (Asparagus racemosus) may be prescribed to address the underlying imbalance in the body.

Heel Fissure in Modern Medicine

In modern medicine, heel fissures are a common condition known as "cracked heels" or "heel fissures." They occur when the skin around the heels becomes dry, thickened, and develops small cracks. Several factors contribute to the development of heel fissures:

Dry Skin: Dry skin is one of the primary causes of heel fissures. Factors such as climate, low humidity, and inadequate hydration can lead to dryness of the skin, making it more prone to cracking.

Excessive Pressure: Standing for long periods, walking barefoot, or wearing open-back shoes can put excessive pressure on the heels, leading to the formation of cracks.

Obesity: Excess body weight can increase pressure on the feet, leading to the development of heel fissures.

Poor Foot Hygiene: Lack of proper foot care, such as not moisturizing the feet regularly or not removing dead skin, can contribute to the development of cracked heels.

Medical Conditions: Certain medical conditions like diabetes, thyroid disorders, or psoriasis can predispose individuals to develop dry, cracked skin, including on the heels.

The management of heel fissures in modern medicine typically includes:
Miniaturization: Applying thick moisturizing creams or ointments to the heels multiple times a day helps to hydrate the skin and soften the cracks.

Exfoliation: Removing dead skin from the heels through gentle exfoliation using a pumice stone or foot file helps to smoothen the skin surface and prevent further cracking.

Foot Soaks: Soaking the feet in warm water for about 10-15 minutes before exfoliation can help to soften the skin and make it easier to remove dead skin cells.

Proper Footwear: Wearing properly fitted shoes with adequate support and cushioning can help to reduce pressure on the heels and prevent further damage.

Medical Treatment: In severe cases or if there is an underlying medical condition, a healthcare professional may prescribe topical medications containing urea or salicylic acid to promote exfoliation and healing of the cracked skin.

Addressing Underlying Conditions: Managing underlying medical conditions like diabetes or thyroid disorders is essential to prevent complications and promote overall foot health.

❖ ❖ ❖ ❖

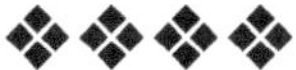 HERPES (विसर्प)

Herpes According to Ayurveda

In Ayurveda, herpes, known as "Visarpa" or "Kshudra Kushta," is described as a viral infection primarily affecting the skin and mucous membranes. According to Ayurvedic principles, herpes is believed to be caused by the aggravation of the Pitta and Kapha doshas, leading to the manifestation of symptoms.

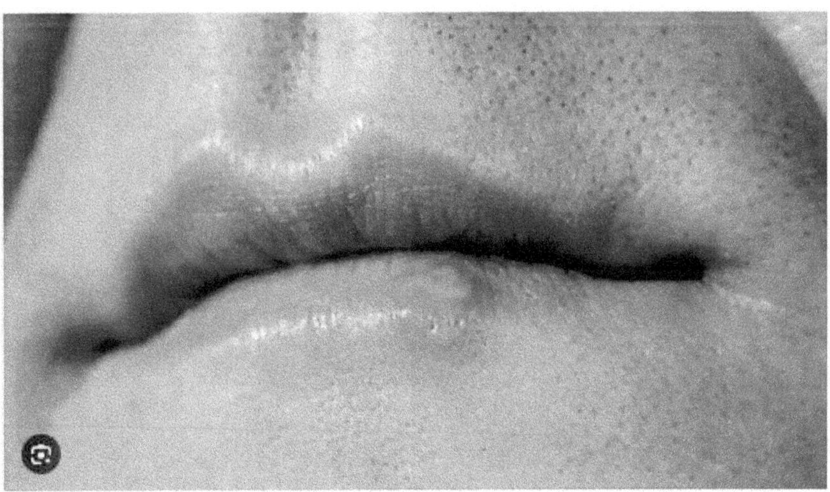

The classical texts of Ayurveda, such as Charaka Samhita and Sushruta Samhita, provide detailed descriptions of herpes and its treatment. According to Ayurveda, herpes is classified into different types based on the doshic involvement and the specific symptoms manifested.

Pitta Type Herpes: This type of herpes is characterized by symptoms such as redness, inflammation, burning sensation, and fever blisters. It is primarily caused by the aggravation of Pitta dosha. Ayurvedic treatments for Pitta type herpes aim to pacify the aggravated Pitta dosha through cooling and soothing therapies.

Kapha Type Herpes: Kapha type herpes is characterized by symptoms such as itching, oozing blisters, and a feeling of heaviness. It occurs due to the vitiation of Kapha dosha. Ayurvedic treatments for Kapha type herpes focus on reducing Kapha accumulation and promoting detoxification.

Vata Type Herpes: Vata type herpes manifests with symptoms such as dryness, cracking of skin, and pain. It is caused by the imbalance of Vata dosha. Ayurvedic treatments for Vata type herpes involve therapies that balance Vata dosha and nourish the affected tissues.

Ayurvedic management of herpes includes a combination of internal medications, external applications, and lifestyle modifications. Some common Ayurvedic herbs and formulations used in the treatment of herpes include:

Neem (Azadirachta Indica): Neem is known for its antiviral and immune-boosting properties. It helps in reducing the severity of herpes symptoms and prevents recurrent outbreaks.

Manjistha (Rubia Cordifolia): Manjistha is a blood-purifying herb that helps in detoxifying the body and promoting skin health. It is beneficial in managing herpes by purifying the blood and reducing inflammation.

Guduchi (Tinospora Cordifolia): Guduchi boosts the immune system and helps the body fight against viral infections, including herpes.

Triphala: Triphala, a combination of three fruits (Amalaki, Bibhitaki, and Haritaki), is known for its detoxifying and rejuvenating properties. It helps in balancing the doshas and promoting overall health.

Chandanasava: Chandanasava is an Ayurvedic tonic that contains Chandan (sandalwood) and other herbs. It helps in reducing inflammation, itching, and burning sensation associated with herpes.

Apart from herbal remedies, Ayurveda emphasizes the importance of maintaining a healthy diet and lifestyle to prevent and manage herpes outbreaks. Avoiding spicy, oily, and acidic foods, practicing good hygiene, managing stress, and getting an adequate amount of sleep are essential aspects of Ayurvedic management of herpes.

Herpes in Modern Medicine

In modern medicine, herpes is a viral infection caused by the herpes simplex virus (HSV). There are two main types of herpes viruses: HSV-1 and HSV-2.

HSV-1: This type of herpes primarily causes oral herpes, including cold sores or fever blisters around the mouth and on the lips. However, it can also cause genital herpes through oral-genital contact.

HSV-2: HSV-2 mainly causes genital herpes, which results in sores and blisters in the genital area. It is primarily transmitted through sexual contact.

Herpes infections are characterized by recurrent outbreaks of painful sores, blisters, and ulcers in the affected areas. The virus remains dormant in the body and can become reactivated, leading to recurrent outbreaks.

Modern Medicine Offers Several Treatment Options For Herpes, Including:

Antiviral Medications: Drugs such as acyclovir, valacyclovir, and famciclovir are commonly prescribed to manage herpes outbreaks. These medications can help reduce the severity and duration of symptoms, as well as decrease the frequency of outbreaks.

Topical Treatments: Antiviral creams and ointments, such as acyclovir cream or penciclovir cream, can be applied directly to the affected areas to help alleviate symptoms and promote healing.

Pain Relief Medications: Over-the-counter pain relievers, such as ibuprofen or acetaminophen, may be recommended to relieve pain and discomfort associated with herpes outbreaks.

Suppressive Therapy: For individuals with frequent or severe herpes outbreaks, doctors may prescribe long-term antiviral therapy to suppress the virus and reduce the frequency of outbreaks. This approach can also help reduce the risk of transmitting the virus to sexual partners.

In addition to medication, practicing safe sex, using condoms during sexual activity, and avoiding sexual contact during outbreaks can help prevent the spread of genital herpes. Regular testing for sexually transmitted infections (STIs) and open communication with sexual partners are also important preventive measures.

While modern medicine does not offer a cure for herpes, antiviral medications and other treatments can help manage symptoms and reduce the frequency of outbreaks, improving the quality of life for individuals affected by the virus.

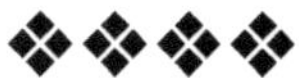

HYPERHIDROSIS (श्वेद आधिक्य)

Hyperhidrosis According to Ayurveda

Hyperhidrosis is primarily associated with an aggravation of Pitta dosha, which governs metabolism and heat regulation in the body. When Pitta becomes imbalanced, it can lead to excessive sweating, especially in the palms, soles, and underarms.

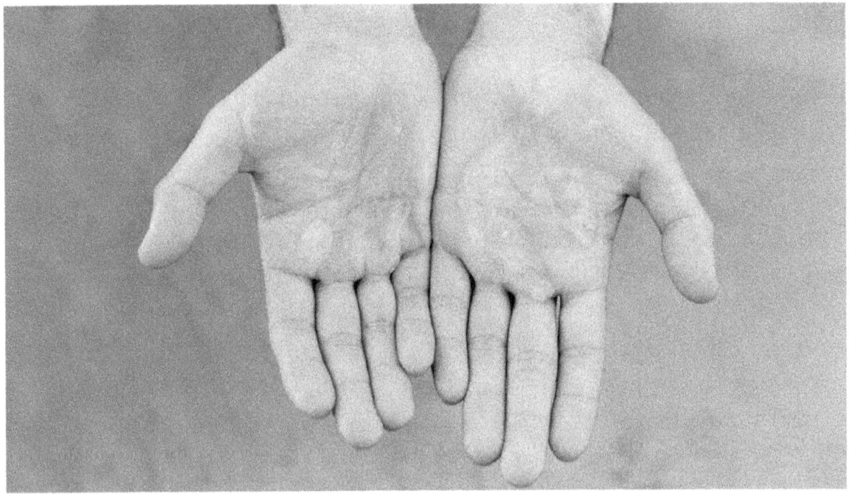

According to Ayurvedic principles, several factors can contribute to the aggravation of Pitta dosha and the manifestation of hyperhidrosis. These include:

Dietary Factors: Consuming excessively spicy, sour, and salty foods can aggravate Pitta dosha. Ayurveda recommends a cooling and Pitta-pacifying diet consisting of sweet, bitter, and astringent tastes to balance Pitta and reduce excessive sweating.

Emotional Factors: Stress, anxiety, and anger are known to increase Pitta in the body, leading to hyperhidrosis. Ayurvedic practices such as meditation, yoga, and pranayama (breathing exercises) are recommended to calm the mind and balance Pitta dosha.

Environmental Factors: Exposure to hot weather, intense sunlight, and high humidity can exacerbate Pitta dosha and worsen hyperhidrosis. Ayurveda advises staying cool and hydrated, avoiding direct sun exposure, and seeking shade during peak hours to prevent excessive sweating.

Lifestyle Factors: Irregular daily routines, excessive physical activity, and inadequate rest can disturb the balance of Pitta dosha and contribute to hyperhidrosis. Following a consistent daily routine, getting enough sleep, and engaging in moderate exercise are essential for maintaining Pitta balance.

Ayurvedic treatment for hyperhidrosis focuses on pacifying Pitta dosha and restoring balance to the body. This may include:

Herbal Remedies: Ayurvedic herbs such as Shatavari, Brahmi, Neem, and Amla are known for their cooling and Pitta-pacifying properties. These herbs can be taken internally or used topically to reduce excessive sweating.

Dietary Modifications: Following a Pitta-pacifying diet that includes cooling foods such as cucumber, coconut, and melons can help balance Pitta dosha and alleviate hyperhidrosis.

Lifestyle Modifications: Practicing stress management techniques, maintaining a regular daily routine, and avoiding triggers that aggravate Pitta dosha are essential for managing hyperhidrosis in Ayurveda.

Panchakarma Therapy: Ayurvedic detoxification therapies such as Panchakarma can help eliminate toxins from the body, balance the doshas, and alleviate symptoms of hyperhidrosis.

Yoga and Meditation: Incorporating yoga asanas (postures) and meditation into daily life can help calm the mind, reduce stress, and balance Pitta dosha, thereby reducing excessive sweating.

Hyperhidrosis in Modern Medicine

Hyperhidrosis, a medical condition characterized by excessive sweating beyond what is necessary for thermoregulation, is studied and treated within modern medicine through various approaches, including diagnosis, management, and treatment options.

Diagnosis: In modern medicine, hyperhidrosis is diagnosed based on medical history, physical examination, and sometimes additional tests such as the starch-iodine test or sweat chloride test. These tests help determine the severity and extent of sweating and rule out underlying medical conditions that may be contributing to the symptoms.

Classification: Hyperhidrosis is classified into two main types: primary and secondary. Primary hyperhidrosis typically affects specific areas of the body, such as the palms, soles, underarms, and face, without an underlying medical cause. Secondary hyperhidrosis is associated with an underlying medical condition or medication use.

Treatment Options:

Topical Treatments: Antiperspirants containing aluminum chloride are commonly used as the first line of treatment for hyperhidrosis. These products work by blocking sweat ducts and reducing sweating in affected areas.

Oral Medications: In some cases, oral medications such as anticholinergics or beta-blockers may be prescribed to reduce sweating. These medications work by blocking the signals that stimulate sweat glands.

Botulinum Toxin Injections: Botulinum toxin injections, commonly known as Botox injections, can be administered to temporarily block the nerves that stimulate sweat glands, effectively reducing sweating in targeted areas. This treatment is particularly effective for axillary hyperhidrosis (excessive sweating in the underarms).

Iontophoresis: This therapy involves passing a mild electric current through water or a wet pad to the affected areas, such as the hands or feet, to temporarily block sweat glands. It is often used for patients with palmar or plantar hyperhidrosis.

Surgery: For severe cases of hyperhidrosis that do not respond to other treatments, surgical procedures such as sympathectomy (endoscopic thoracic sympathectomy or ETS) may be considered. ETS involves cutting or clamping the nerves that control sweating in the affected areas.

Laser Therapy: Laser therapy, such as laser sweat ablation, is a minimally invasive procedure that targets and destroys sweat glands in the underarms, resulting in reduced sweating.

Lifestyle Modifications: Along with medical interventions, lifestyle modifications such as wearing breathable clothing, avoiding triggers that exacerbate sweating (e.g., spicy foods, hot beverages), and practicing stress-reduction techniques can help manage hyperhidrosis symptoms.

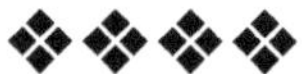

IMPETIGO (पानीवात)

Impetigo According to Ayurveda

Impetigo, known as "पानीवात" in Ayurveda, is a skin infection characterized by red sores that quickly rupture, ooze, and then form a yellowish-brown crust. According to Ayurveda, impetigo is primarily caused by an imbalance of the Pitta and Kapha doshas, leading to the accumulation of toxins (ama) in the body. Here's a detailed essay on impetigo according to Ayurveda:

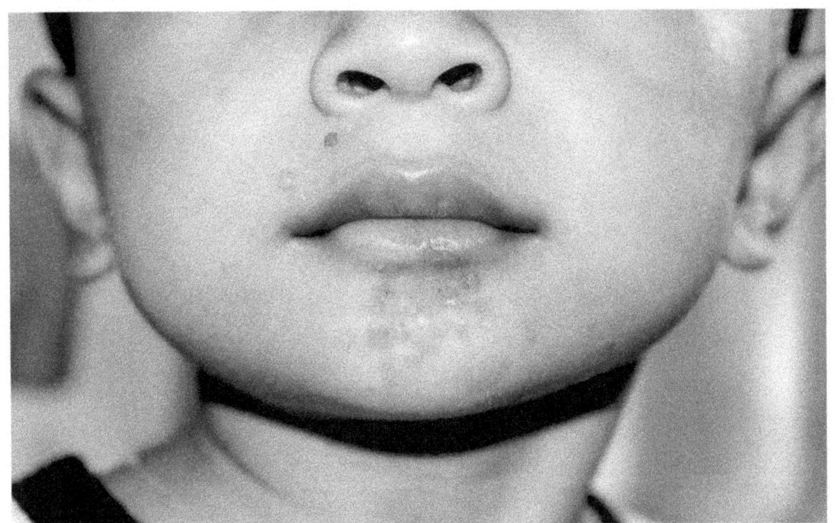

Impetigo, known as पानीवात in Ayurveda, is a common contagious skin infection primarily affecting children but can occur in individuals of any age. It manifests as red sores that rupture, releasing pus-like fluid and forming a crust. In Ayurveda, impetigo is classified under the category of "Kshudra Kushtha," which refers to minor skin diseases.

Etiology (Nidana): According to Ayurveda, impetigo is caused by an imbalance in the Pitta and Kapha doshas. Excessive intake of Pitta-aggravating foods such as spicy, oily, and sour foods, as well as exposure to Kapha-aggravating factors such as cold and damp environments, can predispose an individual to impetigo. Poor hygiene practices, skin injuries, and weakened immunity also contribute to the development of this condition.

Pathogenesis (Samprapti): The imbalance of Pitta and Kapha doshas leads to the accumulation of toxins (ama) in the body. These toxins then localize in the skin, obstructing the microchannels (srotas) and impairing the natural healing mechanisms of the skin. This results in the formation of red, oozing sores characteristic of impetigo.

Clinical Features (Rupa): Impetigo typically presents as clusters of red sores on the face, especially around the nose and mouth, but can also occur on other parts of the body. The sores quickly rupture, releasing a honey-colored fluid that dries to form a yellowish-brown crust. Itching and discomfort are common symptoms associated with impetigo.

Ayurvedic Management (Chikitsa): The treatment approach in Ayurveda aims to rebalance the aggravated doshas, eliminate toxins from the body, and promote skin healing. The following modalities are commonly employed:

Dietary Modification: Avoidance of Pitta and Kapha-aggravating foods such as spicy, oily, and sour foods. Emphasis is placed on consuming cooling and detoxifying foods such as fresh fruits, vegetables, and herbal teas.

Herbal Remedies: Internal administration of herbs with Pitta and Kapha-pacifying properties, such as neem (Azadirachta indica), turmeric (Curcuma longa), and guduchi (Tinospora cordifolia). These herbs help to purify the blood, enhance immunity, and support skin healing.

Topical Applications: Application of herbal pastes or oils containing antimicrobial and wound-healing herbs such as neem, turmeric, and manjistha (Rubia cordifolia) directly to the affected areas. This helps to reduce inflammation, prevent secondary infections, and promote crust formation.

Hygiene Practices: Maintaining proper hygiene is essential to prevent the spread of impetigo. Regular bathing with warm water and gentle cleansing of the affected areas with herbal soaps or decoctions helps to remove crusts and reduce bacterial colonization.

Lifestyle Modification: Avoidance of factors that aggravate Pitta and Kapha doshas, such as excessive sun exposure, stress, and sedentary lifestyle. Engaging in regular physical activity, adequate sleep, and stress-reducing practices such as yoga and meditation promote overall well-being and support skin health.

Impetigo in Modern Medicine

Impetigo is a common bacterial skin infection that can affect people of all ages, characterized by red sores that quickly rupture, ooze, and form crusts. In modern medicine, impetigo is primarily caused by Staphylococcus aureus or Streptococcus pyogenes bacteria

Etiology: The main causative agents of impetigo are Staphylococcus aureus and Streptococcus pyogenes bacteria. These bacteria can enter the skin through breaks or cuts, or they can colonize healthy skin. Factors such as poor hygiene, warm and humid environments, crowded living conditions, and compromised skin barrier function increase the risk of developing impetigo.

Pathogenesis: Upon entering the skin, Staphylococcus aureus and Streptococcus pyogenes bacteria multiply and produce toxins that damage the skin tissue. This leads to the formation of small vesicles or blisters, which quickly rupture, releasing fluid that contains bacteria and inflammatory mediators. The skin lesions then become crusted and may spread to other parts of the body through scratching or contact with contaminated objects.

Clinical Features: Impetigo typically presents as small red papules or vesicles that quickly rupture, forming superficial erosions with a characteristic honey-colored crust. The lesions are often surrounded by redness and may be itchy or painful. Impetigo can occur on any part of the body but is most commonly found on the face, especially around the nose and mouth.

Diagnosis: The diagnosis of impetigo is primarily clinical, based on the characteristic appearance of the skin lesions. Laboratory tests, such as bacterial cultures or polymerase chain reaction (PCR) assays, may be performed to identify the causative bacteria and determine antibiotic susceptibility in cases of recurrent or severe impetigo.

Treatment: The mainstay of treatment for impetigo is topical or oral antibiotics to eradicate the bacterial infection. Topical antibiotics, such as mupirocin or fusidic acid, are typically used for localized, mild cases, while oral antibiotics, such as amoxicillin-clavulanate or cephalexin, may be prescribed for more extensive or severe infections. Good hygiene practices, such as regular handwashing and keeping the affected areas clean and dry, are essential to prevent the spread of impetigo.

Complications: Although impetigo is usually a benign condition, complications such as cellulitis, lymphangitis, and post-streptococcal glomerulonephritis may occur, especially in cases of untreated or inadequately treated infection. Prompt recognition and treatment of impetigo are important to prevent complications and minimize the risk of transmission to others.

Prevention: Preventive measures for impetigo include practicing good hygiene, avoiding contact with infected individuals or contaminated objects, and promptly treating any skin injuries or infections. In certain settings, such as schools or daycare centers, implementing measures to promote hand hygiene and environmental cleanliness can help prevent outbreaks of impetigo.

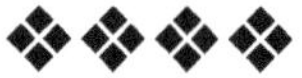

INSECT BITE (कीड़ा काटना)

Insect Bite According to Ayurveda

In Ayurveda, the ancient Indian system of medicine, insect bites are classified under the category of "Visha," which refers to toxins or poisons.

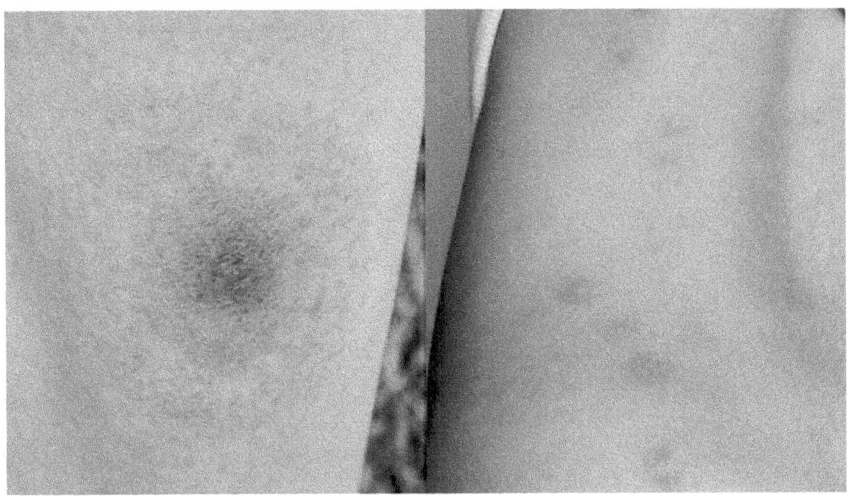

Insect bites, considered as external invasions, disrupt the balance of doshas, leading to discomfort and potential health complications.

Classification of Insect Bites:

Ayurveda categorizes insect bites based on the predominant dosha imbalance they cause and the type of insect involved. For example:

Vata-Predominant Bites: Bites from insects like mosquitoes or flies often result in symptoms related to Vata imbalance, such as itching, dryness, and a feeling of lightness in the affected area.

Pitta-Predominant Bites: Insects like bees, wasps, or fire ants can cause bites that aggravate Pitta dosha, leading to symptoms such as inflammation, redness, and burning sensation at the site of the bite.

Kapha-Predominant Bites: Some insects, like ticks or fleas, may cause Kapha-related symptoms such as swelling, heaviness, and a feeling of coolness in the affected area.

Symptoms of Insect Bites:

The symptoms of insect bites according to Ayurveda may vary depending on the dosha imbalance caused by the bite. Common symptoms include:

- **Itching**
- **Redness**
- **Swelling**
- **Inflammation**
- **Burning sensation**
- **Pain or discomfort**
- **Formation of blisters or rashes**

Ayurvedic Approach to Treating Insect Bites:

Ayurveda emphasizes a holistic approach to treating insect bites, focusing on restoring the balance of doshas and alleviating symptoms naturally. Treatment strategies may include:

Pacifying Dosha Imbalance: Ayurvedic remedies aim to balance the aggravated dosha responsible for the symptoms. For example, Vata-pacifying herbs like licorice or ashwagandha may be used for Vata-related symptoms, while Pitta-pacifying herbs like aloe vera or neem are beneficial for Pitta-related symptoms.

Local Application of Herbal Preparations: Herbal pastes or oils containing cooling and soothing herbs like neem, turmeric, or sandalwood may be applied topically to the affected area to reduce inflammation, itching, and pain.

Internal Medications: Internal herbal formulations or supplements may be prescribed to address systemic imbalances and enhance the body's natural healing process. These may include formulations containing herbs like triphala, guduchi, or guggul.

Dietary and Lifestyle Modifications: Adjustments in diet and lifestyle can help support the body's healing process and prevent future occurrences of insect bites. This may involve consuming cooling and hydrating foods, avoiding spicy or oily foods, and adopting practices that promote relaxation and stress reduction.

Preventive Measures: Ayurveda advocates preventive measures to minimize the risk of insect bites, such as using natural insect repellents, wearing protective clothing, and maintaining cleanliness in living spaces.

Insect Bite in Modern Medicine

In modern medicine, insect bites are typically classified based on the type of insect involved and the reaction they trigger in the body. While the approach to treating insect bites in modern medicine differs from that of Ayurveda, both systems aim to alleviate symptoms and prevent complications.
Insects are ubiquitous in our environment, and their bites can often lead to discomfort, allergic reactions, and in some cases, serious health complications. In modern medicine, the approach to understanding and treating insect bites is grounded in scientific principles and evidence-based.

Classification of Insect Bites:

Modern medicine classifies insect bites based on the type of insect responsible for the bite and the reaction they trigger in the body. Common classifications include:

Mosquito Bites: Mosquitoes are notorious for causing itchy, raised bumps on the skin due to their saliva injected during feeding. In addition to irritation, mosquito bites can transmit diseases such as malaria, dengue fever, and West Nile virus.

Bee and Wasp Stings: Bees and wasps inject venom into the skin when they sting, leading to immediate pain, swelling, and redness at the site of the sting. In individuals with allergies, bee and wasp stings can trigger severe allergic reactions known as anaphylaxis.

Tick Bites: Ticks attach themselves to the skin and feed on blood, potentially transmitting diseases such as Lyme disease, Rocky Mountain spotted fever, and tick paralysis.

Spider Bites: While most spider bites result in mild symptoms such as pain, redness, and swelling, bites from venomous spiders like black widows or brown recluse spiders can cause severe reactions requiring medical attention.

Symptoms of Insect Bites:

The symptoms of insect bites vary depending on the type of insect involved and individual sensitivity. Common symptoms include:

Itching
Pain or Discomfort
Swelling
Redness
Rash or Hives
Localized Heat or Warmth
Formation of Blisters or Pustules

In some cases, insect bites can lead to systemic symptoms such as fever, headache, nausea, and difficulty breathing, especially in individuals with allergies or sensitivities.

Treatment of Insect Bites:

The treatment of insect bites in modern medicine focuses on relieving symptoms and preventing complications. Depending on the severity of the reaction, treatment options may include:

Topical Therapies: Over-the-counter creams, lotions, or ointments containing antihistamines, corticosteroids, or calamine can help reduce itching, inflammation, and discomfort associated with insect bites.

Oral Medications: Oral antihistamines or nonsteroidal anti-inflammatory drugs (NSAIDs) may be prescribed to alleviate itching, pain, and swelling caused by insect bites.

Epinephrine Injection: Individuals with severe allergic reactions to insect stings may carry an epinephrine auto-injector (EpiPen) to administer in case of anaphylaxis, a life-threatening condition requiring immediate medical attention.

Antibiotics: In cases where insect bites become infected due to scratching or secondary bacterial invasion, antibiotics may be prescribed to treat bacterial infections.

Tick Removal: Proper removal of ticks using fine-tipped tweezers and avoiding squeezing or crushing the tick can help prevent the transmission of tick-borne diseases.

Preventive Measures:

Preventing insect bites is key to reducing the risk of associated complications. Modern medicine recommends the following preventive measures:

Using insect repellents containing DEET, picaridin, or oil of lemon eucalyptus
Wearing protective clothing such as long sleeves, pants, and hats
Avoiding areas with high insect activity, especially during dawn and dusk
Checking for ticks after outdoor activities and promptly removing any attached ticks
Seeking medical attention for suspected allergic reactions or unusual symptoms following insect bites

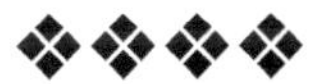

ICHTHYOSIS (इचियोसिस)

Ichthyosis According to Ayurveda

Ichthyosis is a group of genetic skin disorders characterized by dry, scaly skin that resembles fish scales. In Ayurveda, ichthyosis is understood through the lens of doshas (biological energies) and the impact of imbalances on the skin.

According to Ayurveda, ichthyosis primarily stems from an imbalance in the Vata dosha, which governs movement and dryness in the body. When Vata is aggravated, it can lead to excessive dryness in the skin, causing it to become rough and scaly.

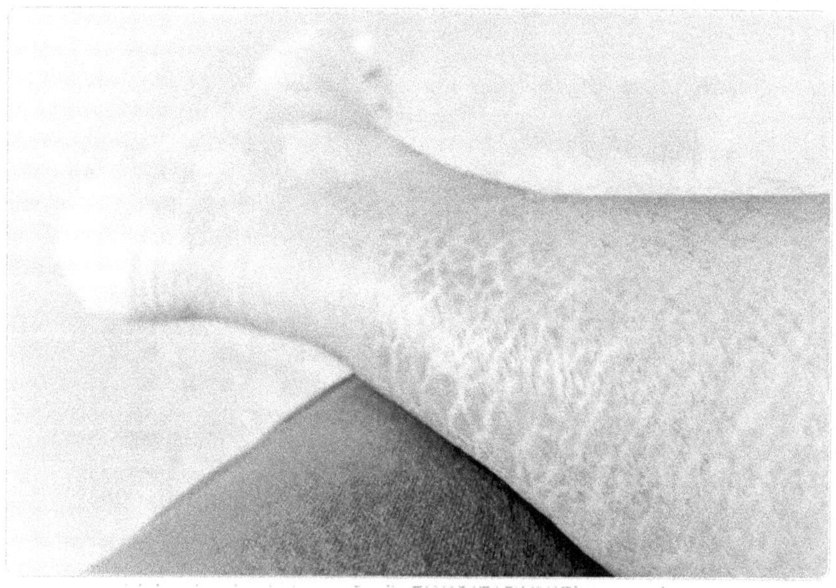

Ayurvedic treatment for ichthyosis aims to pacify the aggravated Vata dosha and restore balance to the skin. This is typically achieved through a combination of dietary modifications, lifestyle changes, and herbal remedies.

Dietary Modifications: Ayurveda emphasizes the importance of a balanced diet to maintain overall health, including skin health. For individuals with ichthyosis, it is recommended to include foods that help pacify Vata dosha and promote skin hydration. This may include warm, moist, and nourishing foods such as cooked grains, soups, steamed vegetables, and healthy fats like ghee and coconut oil.

Lifestyle Changes: Lifestyle factors play a significant role in managing ichthyosis. Ayurveda advises individuals to follow a daily routine (dinacharya) that includes practices to calm Vata dosha, such as regular oil massages (abhyanga) using moisturizing oils like sesame or almond oil. Keeping the skin hydrated by drinking plenty of warm fluids throughout the day is also essential.

Herbal Remedies: Ayurvedic herbs are often used to support skin health and alleviate symptoms of ichthyosis. Some commonly used herbs include:

Shatavari (Asparagus Racemosus): Known for its moisturizing properties, shatavari helps hydrate the skin from within.

Manjistha (Rubia Cordifolia): This herb is believed to cleanse the blood and promote healthy skin by removing toxins from the body.

Neem (Azadirachta Indica): Neem is revered for its anti-inflammatory and antimicrobial properties, which can help reduce inflammation and prevent infections in the affected skin.

Guduchi (Tinospora Cordifolia): Guduchi boosts the immune system and aids in detoxification, supporting overall skin health.

Ayurvedic practitioners may prescribe specific herbal formulations tailored to individual constitution and imbalances to address ichthyosis effectively.

In addition to these measures, stress management techniques, such as yoga, meditation, and pranayama (breathing exercises), can help alleviate stress, which is known to exacerbate Vata imbalances and worsen skin conditions like ichthyosis.

It's important to note that Ayurvedic treatments for ichthyosis should be personalized based on individual constitution, severity of symptoms, and underlying imbalances. Consulting with a qualified Ayurvedic practitioner is recommended to receive tailored guidance and treatment.

Ichthyosis in Modern Medicine

In modern medicine, ichthyosis is classified as a group of genetic skin disorders characterized by dry, scaly skin. These disorders are typically caused by mutations in genes that are involved in the normal shedding of skin cells and maintenance of skin barrier function.

There Are Several Types of Ichthyosis, Including:

Ichthyosis Vulgaris: This is the most common type of ichthyosis, characterized by dry, scaly skin that often develops in childhood and may improve with age.

X-Linked Ichthyosis: This type primarily affects males and is caused by a mutation in the gene responsible for the production of an enzyme called steroid sulfatase.

Lamellar Ichthyosis: This is a more severe form of ichthyosis characterized by thick, plate-like scales covering the body at birth.

Congenital Ichthyosiform Erythroderma (Cie): This is a group of rare genetic disorders characterized by generalized redness and scaling of the skin from birth.

Treatment for Ichthyosis in Modern Medicine

Topical Treatments: Moisturizers and emollients are often prescribed to hydrate the skin and reduce scaling. In more severe cases, topical medications containing keratolytic agents or retinoids may be used to promote shedding of dead skin cells.

Oral Medications: In some cases, oral retinoid may be prescribed to help reduce scaling and improve the appearance of the skin.

Lifestyle Modifications: Practices such as taking short, lukewarm baths, avoiding harsh soaps, and using humidifiers can help alleviate symptoms and prevent skin dryness.

Genetic Counseling: Genetic counseling may be recommended for individuals with ichthyosis and their families to understand the inheritance pattern of the disorder and the risk of passing it on to future generations.

In addition to medical treatment, individuals with ichthyosis may benefit from psychological support to cope with the social and emotional challenges associated with the condition. Support groups and counseling services can provide valuable resources and assistance in managing the psychosocial aspects of living with ichthyosis.

Research into the underlying genetic causes of ichthyosis continues, with the goal of developing more targeted therapies and improving outcomes for affected individuals. Early diagnosis, proper management, and ongoing care are essential for optimizing the quality of life for individuals living with ichthyosis.

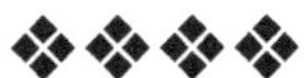

Keloid According to Ayurveda

Keloids, according to Ayurveda, are considered a manifestation of imbalanced doshas, particularly Pitta and Kapha. In Ayurvedic philosophy, keloids are categorized under "kshudra roga" or minor diseases, but their impact on an individual's physical appearance and emotional well-being can be significant.

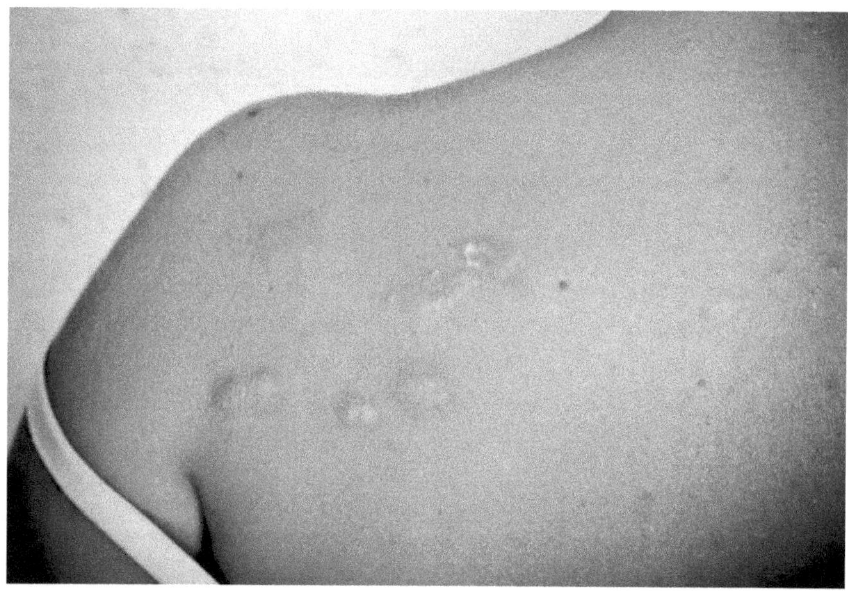

Understanding Keloids in Ayurveda:

Keloids are seen as a result of excessive accumulation of Kapha dosha in the body, leading to the formation of scar tissue that grows beyond the boundaries of the original wound.

Pitta dosha aggravation can also contribute, as it increases inflammation and heat in the affected area, exacerbating the formation of keloids.

Ayurveda emphasizes the importance of considering individual constitution (prakriti) and imbalance (vikriti) in understanding and treating keloids.

Causes of Keloids in Ayurveda:

According to Ayurveda, trauma, burns, surgeries, or any injury that damages the skin and underlying tissues can lead to the formation of keloids.

Genetic predisposition, hormonal imbalances, and certain lifestyle factors that aggravate Pitta and Kapha doshas can also contribute to keloid formation.

Symptoms According to Ayurveda:

Ayurvedic texts describe keloids as raised, firm, nodular growths that extend beyond the original wound site.
They may be accompanied by symptoms such as itching, tenderness, and discoloration of the skin.
Ayurvedic Treatment Approach for Keloids:

Pitta and Kapha Pacifying Diet: Emphasizing foods that balance Pitta and Kapha doshas, such as cooling, bitter, and astringent tastes. This includes fresh fruits and vegetables, whole grains, and avoiding spicy, oily, and processed foods.

Herbal Remedies: Ayurveda offers various herbs with anti-inflammatory, cooling, and wound-healing properties, such as neem, turmeric, aloe vera, and Manjistha (Rubia cordifolia). These can be used internally and externally as pastes or oils.

Panchakarma Therapy: Detoxification therapies like Virechana (therapeutic purgation) and Rakta mokshana (bloodletting) may be recommended to eliminate toxins and balance doshas.

Lifestyle Modifications: Stress management techniques, adequate sleep, and regular exercise are important for maintaining overall health and preventing dosha imbalances.

Preventive Measures:

Avoiding unnecessary trauma to the skin, such as piercings, tattoos, or aggressive skincare treatments.

Maintaining a healthy lifestyle and managing stress to prevent aggravation of Pitta and Kapha doshas.

Keloid in Modern Medicine

In modern medicine, keloids are understood as an abnormal healing response to skin injury, where excessive collagen production leads to the formation of raised, firm, and often disfiguring scars that extend beyond the boundaries of the original wound. Here's a detailed essay on keloids in modern medicine:

Definition and Pathophysiology:

Keloids are benign fibro proliferative growths that occur as a result of abnormal wound healing.
They are characterized by excessive deposition of collagen and other extracellular matrix components.
The exact cause of keloids is not fully understood but is believed to involve genetic predisposition, abnormal wound healing processes, and environmental factors.

Risk Factors:

Genetic Predisposition: Individuals with a family history of keloids are more likely to develop them.

Ethnicity: Certain ethnic groups, particularly those with darker skin tones, are more prone to keloid formation.

Trauma: Any type of skin injury, including surgical incisions, burns, piercings, or acne, can trigger keloid formation.

Hormonal Factors: Keloids may worsen during pregnancy or in individuals with hormonal imbalances.

Clinical Presentation:

Keloids typically present as raised, smooth, shiny nodules or plaques that extend beyond the borders of the original wound.

They may be pink, red, or brown in color and can vary in size and shape.

Symptoms may include itching, pain, and tenderness, which can impact quality of life.

Diagnosis:

Diagnosis of keloids is usually based on clinical examination and patient history.

Skin biopsy may be performed to confirm the diagnosis and rule out other conditions.

Treatment Options:

Surgical Excision: Removing keloids surgically is often ineffective as they have a high recurrence rate.

Corticosteroid Injections: Intralesional corticosteroid injections can help flatten keloids and reduce symptoms.

Cryotherapy: Freezing keloids with liquid nitrogen can sometimes reduce their size and symptoms.
Laser Therapy: Various types of lasers, such as pulsed dye lasers or fractional lasers, may be used to reduce redness and flatten keloids.

Silicone Gel Sheets or Pressure Therapy: These methods can help flatten keloids and improve their appearance.

Radiation Therapy: Radiation may be used as a last resort for recurrent keloids but carries risks of side effects.

Prevention:

Minimizing Trauma to The Skin During Procedures or Surgeries.
Early Intervention with Corticosteroid Injections or Other Treatments for High-Risk Individuals.
Genetic Counseling for Individuals with A Family History of Keloids.
Keloids pose a therapeutic challenge in modern medicine due to their high recurrence rate and limited treatment options. A multimodal approach combining surgical, medical, and laser therapies may be necessary for managing keloids effectively and improving patient outcomes. Continued research into the pathogenesis of keloids and the development of novel treatment modalities are essential for better management of this condition.

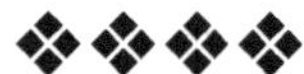

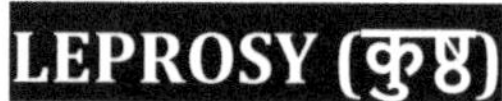

Leprosy According to Ayurveda

In Ayurveda, leprosy, known as "Kushtha," is classified as one of the most severe skin diseases. Ayurvedic texts extensively discuss its etiology, symptoms, classifications, and treatment methods.

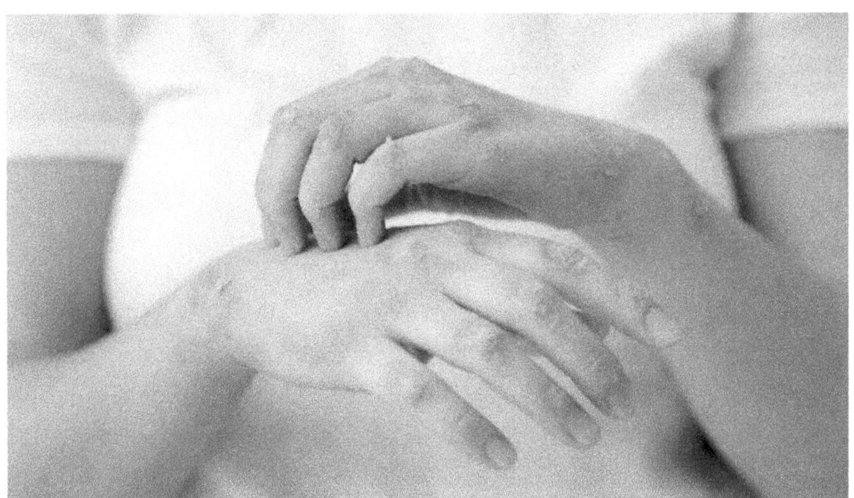

Introduction: Leprosy, or Kushtha, is a chronic infectious disease that primarily affects the skin, nerves, and mucous membranes. It is characterized by disfiguring skin lesions, nerve damage, and progressive debilitation. Ayurveda, the ancient Indian system of medicine, offers a holistic approach to understanding and treating leprosy.

Etiology (Nidana): According to Ayurveda, the imbalance of doshas (biological energies) – Vata, Pitta, and Kapha – plays a crucial role in the development of leprosy. Aggravation of Vata and Kapha doshas, along with impurities in blood (Rakta Dushti), are considered the primary causes of Kushtha.

Types of Kushtha: Ayurveda classifies Kushtha into various types based on clinical manifestations, dosha involvement, and prognosis. The main types include:

Vataja Kushtha: Characterized by dry, scaly skin lesions and severe pain.

Pittaja Kushtha: Exhibits red, inflamed lesions with a burning sensation.

Kaphaja Kushtha: Presents with itching, swelling, and oozing of pus from lesions.

Sannipataja Kushtha: Involves a combination of all three doshas and manifests with diverse symptoms.

Clinical Features (Rupa): Leprosy presents with a wide range of clinical features, including skin lesions, nerve damage, and systemic complications. Common symptoms according to Ayurveda include:

Skin Discoloration: White patches (Sveta Kushtha), reddish-brown patches (Rakta Kushtha), or blackish discoloration (Krishna Kushtha).

Thickened, scaly skin with loss of sensation (Majja Vyapat).
Nerve involvement leading to numbness, weakness, and deformities.
Systemic symptoms like fever, malaise, and weight loss may also occur.

Diagnostic Approach (Nidana Pariksha): Ayurvedic diagnosis of Kushtha involves comprehensive clinical examination, including inspection, palpation, and assessment of doshic imbalance. Pulse diagnosis (Nadi Pariksha) and examination of bodily wastes (Mala Pariksha) are also employed to determine the underlying doshic involvement and severity of the disease.

Treatment Principles (Chikitsa Sutra): Ayurvedic treatment of leprosy aims at correcting doshic imbalance, purifying the blood, and rejuvenating tissues. The treatment modalities include:

Purification Therapies (Shodhana Chikitsa): Panchakarma procedures like Vamana (therapeutic emesis), Virechana (purgation), and Raktamokshana (bloodletting) are performed to eliminate doshic toxins from the body.

Internal Medications (Shamana Chikitsa): Herbal formulations containing anti-inflammatory, antibacterial, and immunomodulatory properties are prescribed to alleviate symptoms and prevent disease progression. Medicinal herbs like Neem (Azadirachta indica), Turmeric (Curcuma longa), and Guduchi (Tinospora cordifolia) are commonly used.

Diet and Lifestyle Modifications: Patients are advised to follow a dosha-balancing diet, avoid incompatible food combinations, and practice stress-reducing techniques like yoga and meditation.

External Therapies: Local application of medicated oils, pastes, and powders helps in soothing skin lesions, reducing inflammation, and promoting healing.

Prognosis (Bhavishya): The prognosis of leprosy in Ayurveda depends on various factors such as the type and stage of the disease, overall health of the patient, and response to treatment.

Leprosy in Modern Medicine

In modern medicine, leprosy, also known as Hansen's disease, is caused by the bacterium Mycobacterium leprae. It primarily affects the skin, peripheral nerves, mucosa of the upper respiratory tract, and eyes. Here's a detailed essay on leprosy in modern medicine:

Leprosy is a chronic infectious disease caused by the slow-growing bacterium Mycobacterium leprae. It primarily affects the skin and peripheral nerves, leading to disfiguring skin lesions, nerve damage, and systemic complications. Leprosy has been a significant public health concern throughout history, but advancements in medical science have improved our understanding of the disease and its management.

Epidemiology: Leprosy is endemic in many countries, particularly in tropical and subtropical regions of Asia, Africa, and Latin America. Despite global efforts to control the disease, leprosy continues to persist in pockets of high endemicity, with approximately 200,000 new cases reported annually worldwide.

Etiology and Pathogenesis: Mycobacterium leprae, the causative agent of leprosy, is an acid-fast, intracellular bacterium that primarily infects macrophages and Schwann cells in the peripheral nervous system. The exact mode of transmission remains uncertain, but prolonged close contact with untreated individuals is considered the primary route of spread. Genetic predisposition, immune status, and environmental factors also influence disease susceptibility and progression.

Clinical Manifestations: Leprosy presents with a spectrum of clinical manifestations ranging from paucibacillary (fewer bacteria) to multibacillary (higher bacterial load) forms. The disease primarily affects the skin and peripheral nerves, leading to the following manifestations:

Skin Lesions: Hypopigmented, erythematous, or nodular skin lesions with decreased sensation.

Nerve Involvement: Peripheral neuropathy causing sensory loss, muscle weakness, and trophic changes like claw hand deformities.

Systemic Complications: Leprosy can affect various organ systems, including eyes, mucous membranes, bones, and testes, leading to blindness, nasal deformities, bone resorption, and infertility.

Diagnostic Approach: Diagnosis of leprosy relies on clinical suspicion, skin biopsy, and bacteriological examination. Skin lesions are examined for characteristic features, and slit skin smears or biopsy specimens are stained and examined under a microscope for acid-fast bacilli. Molecular techniques like polymerase chain reaction (PCR) can also aid in detecting M. leprae DNA.

Treatment and Management: The treatment of leprosy involves multidrug therapy (MDT) regimens recommended by the World Health Organization (WHO). Paucibacillary leprosy is treated with a combination of rifampicin and dapsone, while multibacillary leprosy requires additional clofazimine. Early diagnosis and prompt initiation of MDT can prevent disease progression, reduce transmission, and prevent disabilities.

Prevention and Control: Preventive measures for leprosy include early case detection, contact tracing, and administration of post-exposure prophylaxis to close contacts of confirmed cases. Health education, community awareness programs, and integration of leprosy services into primary healthcare systems are essential for reducing stigma and improving access to care.

Leukoplakia According to Ayurveda

Leukoplakia in Ayurveda, is a condition characterized by white patches on the mucous membranes of the oral cavity, including the tongue, gums, and inner cheeks. In Ayurveda, leukoplakia is primarily understood as a result of vitiation of the doshas, particularly Pitta and Kapha, leading to the accumulation of toxins (ama) in the body.

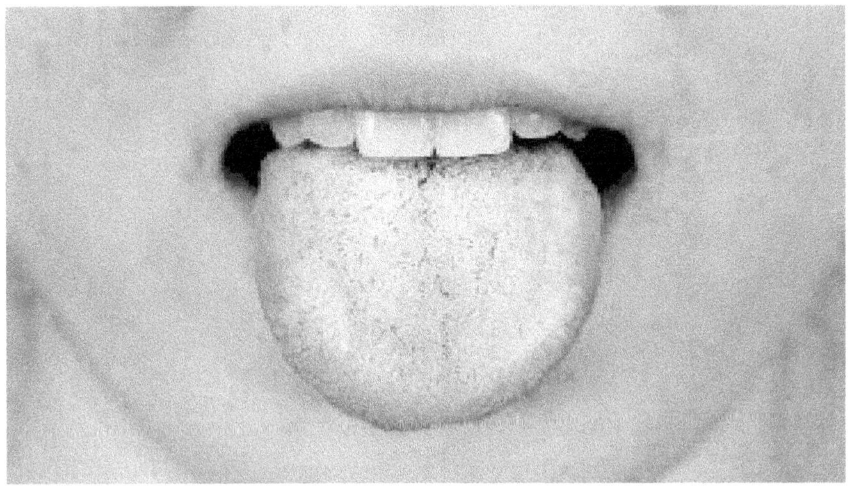

According to Ayurvedic principles, the root cause of leukoplakia lies in the imbalance of Agni (digestive fire), which affects the metabolism and elimination of toxins from the body. When Agni is weak, ama accumulates in the tissues, causing various diseases, including leukoplakia.

Ayurvedic treatment for leukoplakia focuses on restoring the balance of doshas, strengthening Agni, and eliminating ama from the body. This is achieved through a combination of dietary and lifestyle modifications, herbal remedies, and detoxification therapies.

Dietary Recommendations:
Avoid spicy, hot, and acidic foods that can aggravate Pitta dosha.

Include cooling and soothing foods such as fresh fruits, vegetables, and herbal teas.

Drink plenty of water to flush out toxins from the body.

Lifestyle Modifications:

Practice good oral hygiene, including regular brushing and flossing.

Avoid tobacco products, as they are known to worsen leukoplakia.

Practice stress-relieving techniques such as yoga and meditation to balance the mind-body connection.

Herbal Remedies:

Triphala: A combination of three fruits known for its detoxifying properties.

Neem (Azadirachta Indica): Has antibacterial and anti-inflammatory properties that can help in treating oral lesions.

Turmeric (Curcuma Longa): Known for its anti-inflammatory and wound-healing properties.

Detoxification Therapies:

Panchakarma: Ayurvedic detoxification therapies such as Vamana (therapeutic vomiting), Virechana (purgation), and Nasya (nasal administration of medicated oils) may be recommended to eliminate ama from the body.

Gandusha: Oil pulling therapy using medicated oils to cleanse the oral cavity and strengthen the gums.

Rasayana Therapy:

Rasayana herbs such as Ashwagandha (Withania somnifera) and Shatavari (Asparagus racemosus) may be prescribed to rejuvenate the body and improve immunity.

Ayurvedic treatment for leukoplakia aims not only to alleviate symptoms but also to address the underlying imbalance in the body. It emphasizes a holistic approach to health and wellness, focusing on restoring harmony between the mind, body, and spirit.

Leukoplakia in Modern Medicine

Leukoplakia is a condition characterized by white patches on the mucous membranes of the oral cavity, including the tongue, gums, and inner cheeks. In modern medicine, leukoplakia is considered a potentially precancerous lesion, often associated with chronic irritation, such as tobacco use, alcohol consumption, or irritation from dental appliances.

Definition and Causes: Leukoplakia is defined as a white patch or plaque that cannot be scraped off and cannot be clinically diagnosed as any other disease. While the exact cause of leukoplakia is not fully understood, it is believed to be associated with chronic irritation or inflammation of the oral mucosa. Common risk factors include tobacco use, both smoking and smokeless (chewing tobacco), alcohol consumption, chronic irritation from ill-fitting dentures or dental appliances, and viral infections such as human papillomavirus (HPV).

Clinical Presentation: Leukoplakia typically presents as white or grayish patches on the oral mucosa, which may vary in size, shape, and texture. These patches are usually painless but can become irritated or tender if they are rubbed or scraped. In some cases, leukoplakia may be associated with dysplasia, a precancerous change in the cells of the affected tissue.

Diagnosis: Diagnosis of leukoplakia is primarily based on clinical examination. If a white patch or lesion is identified, a biopsy may be performed to rule out other potential causes, such as oral thrush or lichen planus, and to assess for dysplasia or malignant transformation.

Management and Treatment: The management of leukoplakia depends on the underlying cause and the presence of dysplasia or malignant transformation. In cases where leukoplakia is associated with tobacco use or other irritants, cessation of the offending agent is crucial to prevent further progression of the condition. Regular follow-up appointments with a dentist or oral surgeon may be recommended to monitor for changes in the lesion.

If dysplasia or malignant transformation is suspected or confirmed, treatment may involve surgical excision of the lesion or laser therapy to remove the affected tissue. In some cases, topical medications or photodynamic therapy may be used to treat or prevent recurrence of leukoplakia.

Prognosis: The prognosis for leukoplakia depends on various factors, including the size and location of the lesion, the presence of dysplasia or malignant transformation, and the effectiveness of treatment. With early detection and appropriate management, the prognosis for leukoplakia is generally favorable. However, regular monitoring and follow-up care are essential to detect any changes in the lesion and to prevent progression to oral cancer.

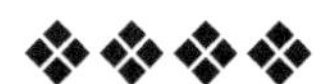

LICHEN PLANUS (लाइकेन प्लानस)

Lichen Planus According to Ayurveda

Lichen Planus is a chronic inflammatory skin condition characterized by the appearance of itchy, reddish-purple, polygonal-shaped papules often with white streaks or scales. In Ayurveda, Lichen Planus is considered a skin disorder primarily caused by an imbalance in the body's doshas, particularly Pitta and Vata.

According to Ayurvedic principles, Lichen Planus manifests when there is an accumulation of ama (toxins) in the body, leading to the disruption of the skin's natural balance. This accumulation can be due to various factors such as improper diet, stress, environmental toxins, and genetic predisposition.

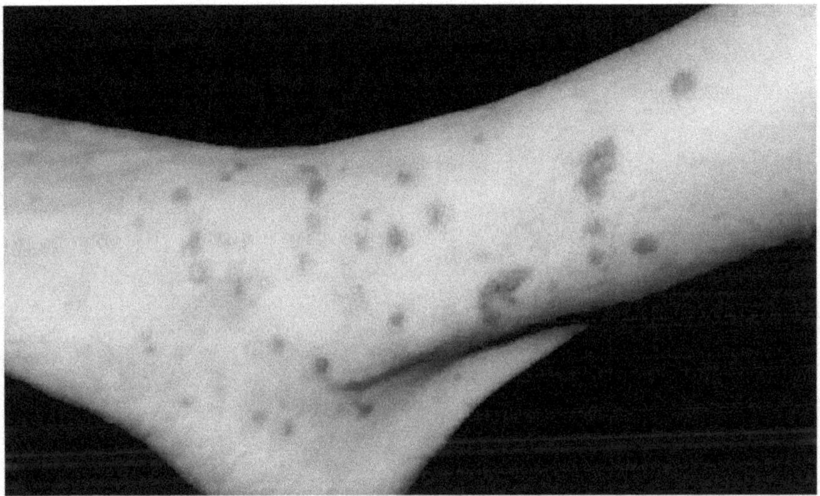

Ayurvedic treatment for Lichen Planus focuses on balancing the doshas, eliminating toxins, and promoting the rejuvenation of the skin. Here are some Ayurvedic approaches commonly used to manage Lichen Planus:

Dietary Modifications: Ayurveda emphasizes the importance of diet in maintaining overall health. Individuals with Lichen Planus are advised to follow a Pitta-pacifying diet, which includes cooling and soothing foods such as fresh fruits, vegetables, whole grains, and herbal teas. Spicy, sour, and acidic foods should be avoided as they can aggravate Pitta dosha.

Herbal Remedies: Ayurvedic herbs are used both internally and externally to treat Lichen Planus. Some commonly prescribed herbs include Neem (Azadirachta indica), Turmeric (Curcuma longa), Aloe Vera (Aloe barbadensis), and Manjistha (Rubia cordifolia). These herbs possess anti-inflammatory, antimicrobial, and detoxifying properties that help to reduce inflammation and promote healing of the skin lesions.

Detoxification Therapies: Panchakarma, the detoxification therapy in Ayurveda, is often recommended for individuals with chronic skin disorders like Lichen Planus. Panchakarma procedures such as Virechana (therapeutic purgation) and Rakta Mokshana (bloodletting) help to eliminate toxins from the body, thereby reducing the severity of symptoms.

Stress Management: Stress is known to exacerbate skin conditions like Lichen Planus. Ayurveda emphasizes the importance of stress management techniques such as yoga, meditation, and pranayama (breathing exercises) to calm the mind and reduce stress levels, which in turn can help improve skin health.

Lifestyle Modifications: Adopting a healthy lifestyle is crucial for managing Lichen Planus. This includes getting an adequate amount of sleep, maintaining proper hygiene, avoiding excessive sun exposure, and staying hydrated.

External Therapies: External applications such as herbal oils, pastes, and ointments are used to soothe the skin, reduce itching, and promote healing of the lesions. Ayurvedic oils containing ingredients like Neem, Manjistha, and Chandan (Sandalwood) are commonly used for topical application.

It's important to note that Ayurvedic treatment for Lichen Planus should be personalized according to an individual's constitution (Prakriti) and specific imbalances. Consulting with a qualified Ayurvedic practitioner is recommended to receive tailored treatment and guidance for managing Lichen Planus effectively while addressing the root cause of the condition.

Lichen Planus in Modern Medicine

In modern medicine, Lichen Planus is recognized as a chronic inflammatory skin condition that can affect various parts of the body, including the skin, mucous membranes, nails, and hair follicles. While the exact cause of Lichen Planus is not fully understood, it is believed to involve an abnormal immune response, genetic factors, and possible triggers such as certain medications, infections, or chemicals.

Symptoms: Lichen Planus typically presents as itchy, reddish-purple, flat-topped papules that may have a shiny appearance. These papules can coalesce to form patches or plaques and often have fine white lines or scales. In addition to the skin, Lichen Planus can affect mucous membranes, causing lesions in the mouth (oral Lichen Planus), genitals, scalp, and nails.

Diagnosis: Diagnosis of Lichen Planus is usually based on the clinical appearance of the lesions. A skin biopsy may be performed to confirm the diagnosis and rule out other skin conditions with similar presentations. In cases of oral Lichen Planus, a biopsy or clinical examination by a dentist or oral pathologist may be necessary.

Treatment: Treatment for Lichen Planus aims to alleviate symptoms, reduce inflammation, and prevent complications. Treatment options may include:

Topical Corticosteroids: Topical corticosteroid creams or ointments are commonly prescribed to reduce inflammation and itching associated with Lichen Planus lesions.

Oral Medications: In cases of widespread or severe Lichen Planus, oral medications such as corticosteroids, retinoids, or immunosuppressants may be prescribed to control symptoms and suppress the immune response.
Phototherapy: Light therapy, such as narrowband ultraviolet B (UVB) phototherapy, may be used to treat resistant cases of Lichen Planus by reducing inflammation and promoting healing of the skin lesions.

Oral Rinses: For oral Lichen Planus, mouthwashes or oral rinses containing corticosteroids, antifungal agents, or calcineurin inhibitors may be recommended to alleviate symptoms and reduce inflammation in the mouth.

Lifestyle Modifications: Avoiding potential triggers such as certain medications, dental materials, or allergens, as well as practicing good oral hygiene, may help manage Lichen Planus and prevent flare-ups.

Long-Term Management: Lichen Planus is a chronic condition that may recur intermittently over time. Long-term management may involve regular follow-up appointments with a dermatologist or other healthcare provider to monitor the condition, adjust treatment as needed, and address any complications such as scarring or pigmentary changes.

Complications: Although Lichen Planus is not contagious and rarely leads to serious health problems, complications such as secondary bacterial or fungal infections, scarring, and changes in skin pigmentation may occur, especially if the lesions are scratched or irritated.

Overall, while there is no cure for Lichen Planus, modern medical treatments can effectively manage symptoms and improve quality of life for individuals affected by this condition. Close collaboration between patients and healthcare providers is essential to develop a personalized treatment plan that addresses the specific needs and concerns of each individual.

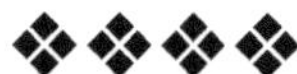

LIPOMA (चर्बी की गांठ)

Lipoma According to Ayurveda

Lipoma, a benign tumor composed of adipose tissue, is viewed in Ayurveda as an imbalance in the body's fat metabolism, primarily involving the Kapha dosha. Ayurveda, an ancient system of medicine originating from India, offers a holistic approach to understanding and treating lipomas.

According to Ayurveda, lipomas are primarily caused by an imbalance in the Kapha dosha, which governs the qualities of heaviness, stability, and lubrication in the body. When Kapha becomes aggravated due to factors such as improper diet, sedentary lifestyle, or genetic predisposition, it can lead to the formation of excess adipose tissue, manifesting as lipomas.

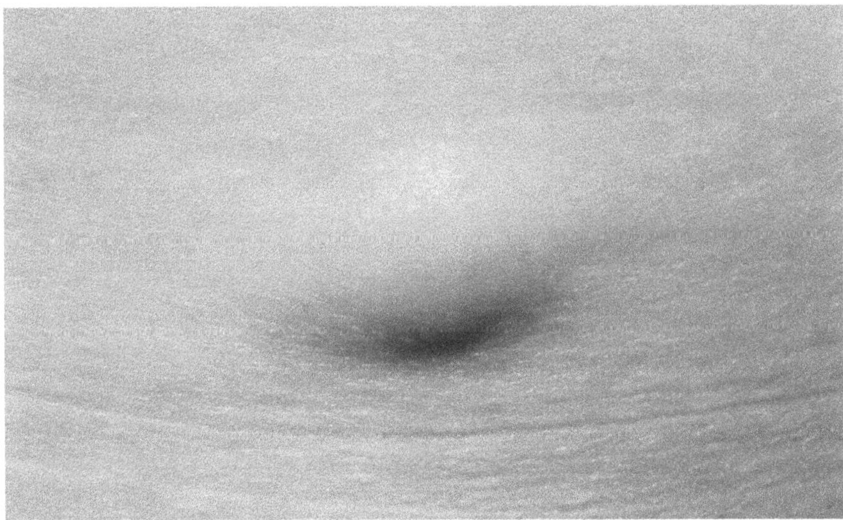

In Ayurveda, the treatment of lipomas aims to pacify the aggravated Kapha dosha and restore balance to the body. This involves a combination of dietary modifications, lifestyle changes, herbal remedies, detoxification therapies, and rejuvenating practices.

Dietary Modifications: Ayurveda emphasizes the importance of following a Kapha-pacifying diet to reduce the accumulation of fatty tissue. This includes consuming warm, light, and dry foods while avoiding heavy, oily, and sweet foods. Incorporating spices such as ginger, turmeric, and cumin can help stimulate digestion and metabolism, thereby reducing Kapha accumulation.

Lifestyle Changes: Leading a sedentary lifestyle can contribute to the accumulation of Kapha and exacerbate the formation of lipomas. Regular exercise, especially activities that promote sweating and detoxification, such as yoga, brisk walking, or aerobic exercises, can help balance the Kapha dosha and prevent the formation of lipomas.

Herbal Remedies: Ayurvedic herbs with properties that reduce Kapha and promote fat metabolism can be beneficial in treating lipomas. Some commonly used herbs include Triphala (a combination of three fruits), Guggulu (Commiphora mukul), Punarnava (Boerhavia diffusa), and Varuna (Crataeva nurvala). These herbs can be taken internally or applied topically in the form of pastes or oils.

Detoxification Therapies: Ayurvedic therapies such as Panchakarma, which includes procedures like Vamana (therapeutic vomiting), Virechana (purgation), and Basti (enema), are effective in detoxifying the body and eliminating excess Kapha. These therapies help remove accumulated toxins and restore balance to the doshas, thereby reducing the size and number of lipomas.

Rejuvenating Practices: Ayurveda also recommends practices that promote overall health and vitality, such as meditation, pranayama (breath control exercises), and Abhyanga (self-massage with herbal oils). These practices help improve circulation, stimulate the lymphatic system, and enhance the body's natural healing mechanisms, which can aid in the treatment of lipomas.

Lipoma in Modern Medicine

In modern medicine, a lipoma is a benign tumor composed of adipose (fat) tissue. It typically presents as a soft, movable lump under the skin, most commonly found on the torso, neck, upper thighs, and armpits. While lipomas are generally harmless and rarely develop into cancer, they can cause discomfort or cosmetic concerns depending on their size and location.

The exact cause of lipomas is not fully understood, but they are believed to result from an overgrowth of fat cells. Some factors that may contribute to their development include:

Genetics: Lipomas often run in families, suggesting a genetic predisposition to their formation.

Age: Lipomas are more common in adults between the ages of 40 and 60, although they can occur at any age.

Gender: Men are slightly more likely to develop lipomas than women.

Obesity: While not all lipomas are associated with obesity, there may be a correlation between excess body fat and the development of lipomas.

In modern medicine, the diagnosis of a lipoma is usually based on its appearance and feel during a physical examination. In some cases, imaging tests such as ultrasound, MRI, or CT scans may be used to confirm the diagnosis or evaluate the size and location of the lipoma.

Treatment of lipomas in modern medicine is typically not necessary unless they cause symptoms such as pain, tenderness, or restricted movement, or if they are cosmetically bothersome. Options for treatment may include:

Surgical Removal: If a lipoma is causing symptoms or cosmetic concerns, it can be surgically removed through a minor outpatient procedure. This involves making an incision in the skin and excising the lipoma along with its capsule.

Liposuction: In some cases, liposuction may be used to remove larger lipomas. This technique involves inserting a thin tube (cannula) into the lipoma and suctioning out the fatty tissue.

Steroid Injections: Injections of corticosteroids into the lipoma may help shrink its size, although this treatment is not always effective and may need to be repeated.

Observation: If a lipoma is small, painless, and not causing any symptoms, it may be left untreated and monitored over time.

Overall, the management of lipomas in modern medicine focuses on relieving symptoms and addressing cosmetic concerns, rather than preventing their occurrence or addressing underlying imbalances in the body's metabolism. However, research into the genetic and molecular mechanisms underlying lipoma development may lead to new insights and treatment approaches in the future.

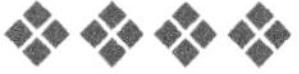

LUPUS (ल्युपस)

Lupus According to Ayurveda

In Ayurveda, Lupus is viewed as a disorder primarily caused by the vitiation of the Vata and Rakta (blood) doshas. It manifests as an autoimmune condition characterized by inflammation, pain, and tissue damage.

Lupus is a chronic autoimmune disorder that affects multiple systems of the body, primarily targeting the joints, skin, kidneys, and other organs. In Ayurveda, it is classified under the broader category of "Vata disorders" due to its predominant involvement of the Vata dosha, which governs movement and communication in the body.

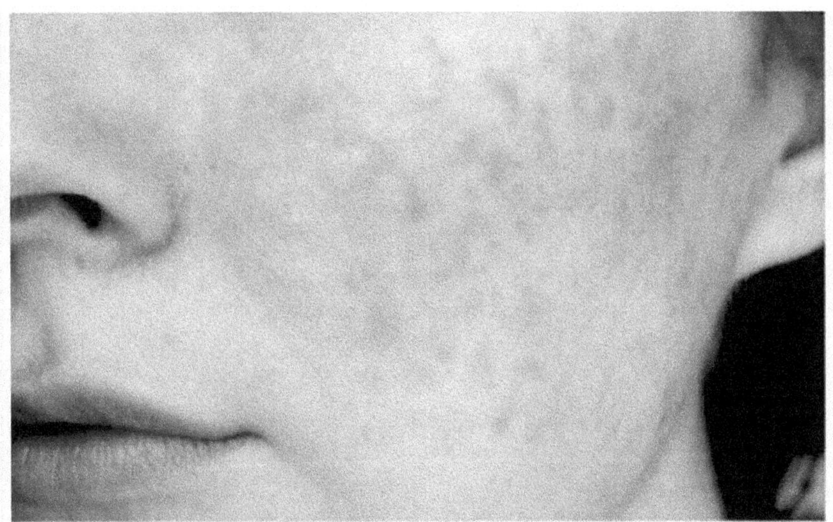

According to Ayurvedic principles, the main causative factors of Lupus include dietary indiscretions, suppression of natural urges, excessive physical and mental stress, and genetic predisposition. These factors disrupt the balance of the Vata dosha and lead to the accumulation of toxins (ama) in the body, particularly in the blood (Rakta dhatu) and joints (Sandhi).

The onset of Lupus is often characterized by symptoms such as joint pain, swelling, stiffness, fatigue, skin rashes, fever, and malaise. Ayurveda emphasizes the importance of identifying the underlying imbalances in each individual's constitution (Prakriti) and addressing them through personalized treatment approaches.

The treatment of Lupus in Ayurveda aims to pacify the aggravated Vata dosha, eliminate toxins from the body, and restore balance to the affected tissues and organs. This holistic approach typically involves a combination of dietary modifications, lifestyle changes, herbal remedies, detoxification therapies, and stress management techniques.

Dietary recommendations for individuals with Lupus focus on consuming warm, easily digestible foods that pacify Vata dosha, such as cooked vegetables, whole grains, lentils, and herbal teas. Avoidance of spicy, fried, and processed foods is also advised to prevent further aggravation of inflammation.

Herbal remedies play a crucial role in managing Lupus symptoms and promoting overall health and well-being. Ayurvedic herbs like Ashwagandha, Guduchi, Turmeric, Triphala, and Guggul are commonly used for their anti-inflammatory, immunomodulatory, and detoxifying properties. These herbs help strengthen the immune system, reduce inflammation, and support the body's natural healing processes.

Detoxification therapies, such as Panchakarma, are recommended to eliminate ama (toxins) from the body and restore balance to the doshas. Panchakarma treatments like Virechana (therapeutic purgation) and Basti (medicated enema) are particularly beneficial for cleansing the blood and rejuvenating the tissues.

In addition to herbal remedies and detoxification therapies, lifestyle modifications are essential for managing Lupus in Ayurveda. Stress management techniques, including yoga, meditation, and breathing exercises, help reduce the impact of psychological stress on the body and promote relaxation and emotional well-being.

Lupus in Modern Medicine

Lupus, known as "ल्युपस" (Lupus) in Hindi, is a complex autoimmune disease that affects various parts of the body, including the skin, joints, kidneys, heart, lungs, brain, and blood cells. In modern medicine, Lupus is considered a chronic inflammatory condition characterized by periods of flare-ups and remission.

The exact cause of Lupus is not fully understood, but it is believed to involve a combination of genetic, environmental, and hormonal factors. Some triggers, such as infections, sunlight, certain medications, and hormonal changes, can activate the immune system in genetically predisposed individuals, leading to inflammation and tissue damage.

The hallmark feature of Lupus is the production of autoantibodies, which mistakenly target and attack healthy tissues and organs, resulting in inflammation and damage. This autoimmune response can manifest in a variety of symptoms, including:

Joint Pain and Swelling (Arthritis)

Skin rashes, such as the characteristic butterfly-shaped rash on the face

Fatigue
Fever
Photosensitivity

Kidney problems, such as proteinuria and nephritis
Neurological symptoms, including headaches, seizures, and cognitive dysfunction

Cardiovascular complications, such as pericarditis and myocarditis

Blood disorders, such as anemia, leukopenia, and thrombocytopenia

Diagnosing Lupus can be challenging due to its variable presentation and overlapping symptoms with other autoimmune and inflammatory conditions. Healthcare providers typically rely on a combination of clinical symptoms, laboratory tests (such as antinuclear antibody testing), imaging studies, and organ biopsies to confirm the diagnosis and assess disease activity.

Treatment for Lupus aims to manage symptoms, prevent flare-ups, and minimize organ damage. This often involves a multidisciplinary approach, including medications, lifestyle modifications, and regular monitoring. Commonly prescribed medications for Lupus include:

Nonsteroidal Anti-Inflammatory Drugs (Nsaids) To Relieve Pain and Inflammation

Antimalarial drugs, such as hydroxychloroquine, to reduce disease activity and protect against skin and joint symptoms

Corticosteroids to suppress the immune system and reduce inflammation during flare-ups

Immunosuppressive drugs, such as methotrexate, azathioprine, mycophenolate mofetil, and cyclophosphamide, to control disease activity and prevent organ damage

Biologic therapies, such as rituximab and belimumab, to target specific components of the immune system involved in Lupus pathogenesis

In addition to medication, lifestyle modifications, such as sun protection, regular exercise, stress management, and a healthy diet, can help improve overall health and well-being in individuals with Lupus.

Despite advances in diagnosis and treatment, Lupus remains a chronic condition with no cure. However, with early diagnosis, prompt treatment, and ongoing medical care, many people with Lupus can effectively manage their symptoms and lead fulfilling lives.

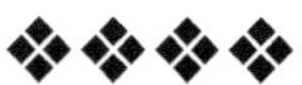

MELASMA (छाइयाँ)

Melasma According to Ayurveda

Melasma, known as "छाइयाँ" in Ayurveda, is a common skin condition characterized by hyperpigmentation, typically appearing as brown or grayish patches on the face. According to Ayurveda, melasma is primarily a result of aggravated Pitta dosha, which is responsible for the body's metabolic processes and governs the skin's complexion. However, imbalances in other doshas, namely Vata and Kapha, can also contribute to its manifestation.

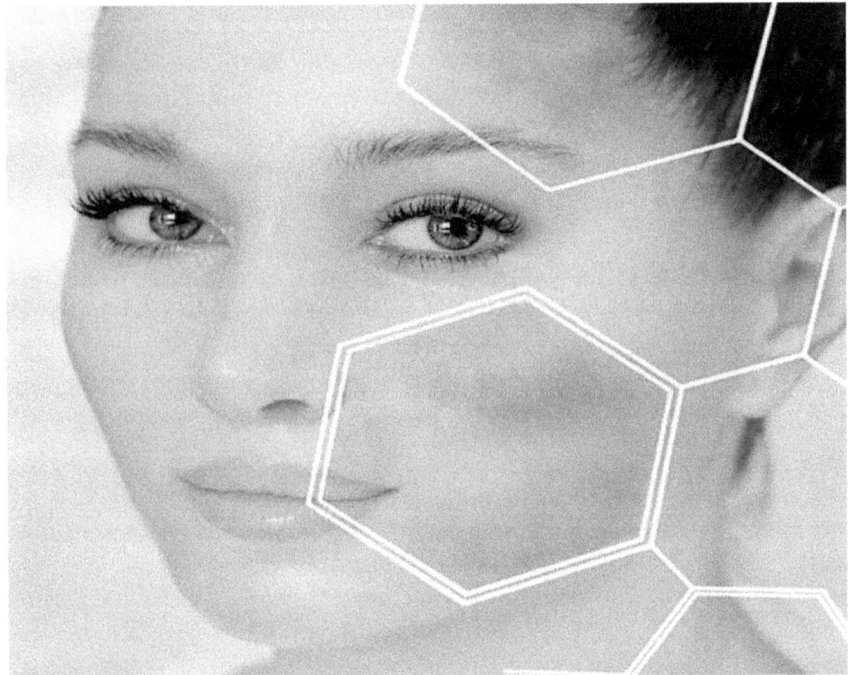

Ayurveda views melasma as a result of internal imbalances, often stemming from dietary habits, lifestyle choices, hormonal fluctuations, and stress. Ayurvedic practitioners emphasize the importance of addressing the root cause of the condition rather than merely treating its symptoms.

Dosha Imbalance: According to Ayurveda, an aggravated Pitta dosha is the primary culprit behind melasma. Pitta governs the metabolic processes in the body and is associated with heat, transformation, and digestion. Excessive intake of Pitta-aggravating foods such as spicy, oily, and acidic foods, as well as exposure to excessive heat and stress, can exacerbate Pitta dosha imbalance, leading to skin issues like melasma.

Ama Formation: Ayurveda also highlights the role of ama, or toxins, in the development of melasma. Poor digestion and metabolism can lead to the accumulation of ama in the body, which in turn can manifest as skin disorders like melasma. Ama disrupts the normal functioning of the body's tissues and channels, including those responsible for maintaining skin health.

Liver Health: The liver plays a crucial role in detoxification according to Ayurveda. An impaired liver function can lead to the accumulation of toxins in the body, further exacerbating Pitta imbalance and contributing to the development of melasma. Therefore, Ayurvedic treatment often includes measures to support liver health and enhance its detoxification functions.

Diet and Lifestyle: Ayurveda emphasizes the importance of a balanced diet and lifestyle to prevent and manage melasma. Pitta-pacifying foods such as cooling fruits and vegetables, whole grains, and herbal teas can help alleviate Pitta imbalance. Additionally, practicing stress-reducing techniques such as yoga, meditation, and pranayama can help calm the mind and balance the doshas.

Herbal Remedies: Ayurveda offers various herbal remedies for treating melasma both internally and externally. Internal remedies may include herbs such as Aloe vera, Neem, Manjistha, and Turmeric, which help purify the blood, cool Pitta, and promote skin health. External treatments often involve the application of herbal pastes or oils containing ingredients like Chandan (Sandalwood), Yashtimadhu (Licorice), and Kumari (Aloe vera) to lighten pigmentation and nourish the skin.

Detoxification Therapies: Ayurvedic detoxification therapies, known as Panchakarma, can also be beneficial in managing melasma. These therapies aim to eliminate ama and rebalance the doshas through procedures such as Virechana (therapeutic purgation) and Raktamokshana (bloodletting). However, these therapies should be performed under the guidance of a qualified Ayurvedic practitioner.

Melasma in Modern Medicine

Melasma, known as "छाइयाँ" in Hindi, is a common skin condition characterized by hyperpigmentation, typically appearing as brown or grayish patches on the face. In modern medicine, melasma is understood to be a complex condition influenced by various factors, including genetics, hormonal changes, exposure to ultraviolet (UV) radiation, and certain medications.

Hormonal Influences: Hormonal changes, particularly during pregnancy or while taking hormonal trigger the development of melasma. This is why melasma is often referred to as "the mask of pregnancy." Fluctuations in estrogen and progesterone levels can stimulate the production of melanin, the pigment responsible for skin color, leading to hyperpigmentation in certain areas of the face.

Uv Exposure: Exposure to sunlight, specifically to ultraviolet A (UVA) and ultraviolet B (UVB) rays, Is a significant risk factor for melasma. UV radiation stimulates the production of melanin and can exacerbate existing hyperpigmentation. Melasma tends to worsen with sun exposure, which is why sun protection, including the use of broad-spectrum sunscreen and protective clothing, is crucial for preventing and managing the condition.

Genetic Predisposition: There is evidence to suggest that genetics plays a role in the development of melasma. Individuals with a family history of the condition are more likely to develop it themselves. Specific genetic factors related to melanin production and distribution may contribute to an individual's susceptibility to melasma.

Skin Type: Certain skin types, particularly those with more melanin-rich skin (Fitzpatrick skin types III-VI), are more prone to developing melasma.

Individuals with darker skin tones have a higher concentration of melanin, which can lead to more pronounced hyperpigmentation.

Other Factors: Other factors that may contribute to the development of melasma include certain medications (e.g., hormonal therapies, antiseizure medications), thyroid disorders, and cosmetics or skincare products that irritate the skin.

Treatment Options: Treatment for melasma typically involves a combination of topical agents, such as hydroquinone, retinoids, corticosteroids, and kojic acid, which help lighten hyperpigmented areas and regulate melanin production. Procedures like chemical peels, microdermabrasion, and laser therapy may also be recommended to improve skin tone and texture. Additionally, strict sun protection measures are essential to prevent further darkening of the affected areas.

Maintenance and Prevention: While treatments can help improve melasma, the condition often requires long-term management and maintenance. Sun protection remains a cornerstone of melasma management, along with the consistent use of prescribed topical agents and avoidance of known triggers. In some cases, melasma may recur despite treatment, requiring ongoing monitoring and adjustment of management strategies.

In summary, melasma is a multifactorial condition influenced by hormonal, genetic, environmental, and lifestyle factors. Understanding these factors is crucial for effective management and prevention. Treatment approaches in modern medicine focus on addressing the underlying causes of melasma, regulating melanin production, and protecting the skin from further damage.

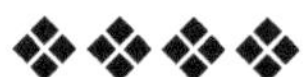

MOLES (तिलकालक)

Moles According to Ayurveda

Moles, known as "तिलकालक" (Tilakalaka) in Ayurveda, hold significance beyond mere skin markings. In Ayurvedic philosophy, moles are believed to be indicative of one's health and personality traits, influenced by doshas (biological energies) - Vata, Pitta, and Kapha.

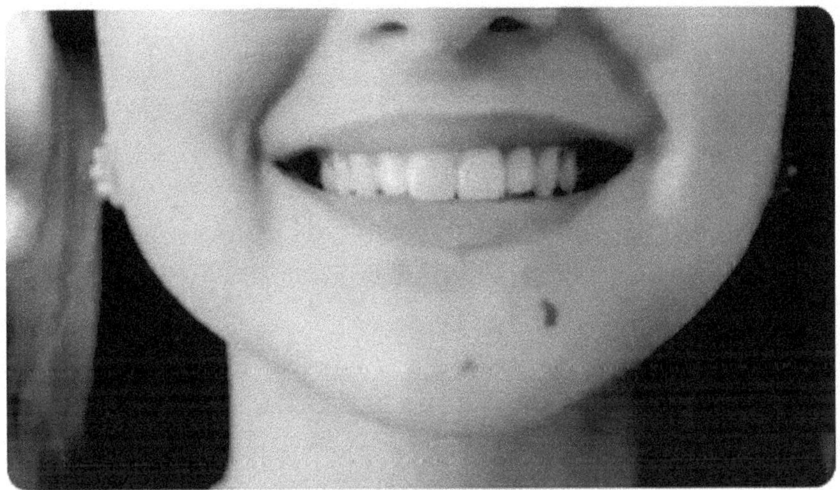

Understanding Moles in Ayurveda

In Ayurveda, the body is viewed as a microcosm of the universe, with each part reflecting the balance or imbalance of the doshas. Moles, or Tilakalaka, are considered to be a manifestation of the body's internal state, serving as markers that reveal underlying health conditions and psychological tendencies.

Classification of Moles

Ayurveda categorizes moles based on their location, size, color, and texture, correlating each characteristic with specific doshic imbalances and their corresponding effects on an individual's well-being.

Location: Moles appearing on different parts of the body are believed to signify various aspects of one's health and personality. For instance, moles on the face may indicate specific organ imbalances, while those on the limbs might suggest issues related to mobility or circulation.

Size: The size of a mole is linked to the intensity of the doshic influence it represents. Larger moles may signify more significant imbalances, while smaller ones could indicate milder disturbances.

Color: Ayurveda associates different colors of moles with specific doshas. Dark moles are often associated with Pitta dosha, while lighter moles may relate to Vata or Kapha doshas.

Texture: The texture of a mole can provide further insights into its nature. Smooth moles are considered benign, while rough or irregular ones may suggest underlying health issues.

Interpreting Moles

Ayurvedic practitioners analyze moles holistically, considering their physical attributes alongside an individual's constitutional doshic makeup and current health status. Through careful observation and assessment, they can decipher the messages encoded in these skin markings.

Health Indicators: Moles are viewed as reflections of internal imbalances, offering valuable clues about potential health issues such as digestive disorders, hormonal imbalances, or metabolic disturbances. By identifying and addressing the root causes behind these imbalances, Ayurvedic remedies aim to restore harmony to the body and promote overall well-being.

Psychological Insights: In addition to their physiological significance, moles are believed to hold psychological implications. Ayurveda suggests that certain mole patterns may correspond to specific personality traits or emotional tendencies, providing insight into an individual's mental and emotional constitution.

Ayurvedic Remedies For Moles

Ayurveda emphasizes a holistic approach to health and wellness, advocating for personalized treatments that address the root cause of imbalances rather than merely alleviating symptoms. Depending on the nature of the mole and the underlying doshic influences, treatment modalities may include:

Dietary Modifications: Adjusting one's diet according to their dominant dosha(s) can help restore balance and prevent the formation of new moles. Incorporating nourishing foods and herbs that pacify aggravated doshas can support skin health and promote detoxification.

Herbal Therapies: Ayurvedic herbs such as neem, turmeric, and manjistha are renowned for their purifying and skin-healing properties. Herbal formulations tailored to individual doshic imbalances can help address skin issues, including the appearance of moles.

Lifestyle Modifications: Adopting lifestyle practices that promote doshic balance, such as regular exercise, adequate sleep, and stress management techniques, can contribute to healthy skin and overall well-being.

Ayurvedic Treatments: External therapies like abhyanga (oil massage), udvartana (herbal scrub), and lepa (herbal paste application) may be recommended to nourish the skin, improve circulation, and support the natural healing process.

Moles in Modern Medicine

In modern medicine, moles, medically known as melanocytic nevi, are viewed primarily as benign skin growths composed of melanocytes, the pigment-producing cells in the skin. While they can vary in size, color, and texture, moles are generally considered harmless unless they exhibit certain concerning features such as asymmetry, irregular borders, multiple colors, or changes in size or shape, which may indicate the possibility of skin cancer, particularly melanoma.

Characteristics Of Moles

Development: Moles typically develop during childhood and adolescence, although they can appear at any age. They often result from a localized proliferation of melanocytes in response to sun exposure or genetic predisposition.

Appearance: Moles can range in color from tan to dark brown and may be flat or raised. They are usually round or oval-shaped and have smooth borders.

Distribution: Moles can occur anywhere on the body, including the face, trunk, limbs, and mucous membranes. Some individuals may have only a few moles, while others may have numerous moles covering their skin.

Risk Factors: While most moles are benign, certain factors, such as a family history of melanoma, fair skin, and excessive sun exposure, can increase the risk of developing abnormal or cancerous moles.

Evaluation And Management

Skin Examination: Dermatologists typically perform thorough skin examinations to assess the characteristics of moles and identify any features suggestive of skin cancer. This may involve visual inspection and, in some cases, dermoscopy, a non-invasive imaging technique that allows for magnified examination of skin lesions.

Biopsy: If a mole exhibits suspicious features, a dermatologist may recommend a biopsy, which involves removing a small sample of tissue for histological examination under a microscope to determine whether the mole is cancerous or benign.

Treatment: Most moles do not require treatment unless they pose a cosmetic concern or exhibit suspicious features. Options for mole removal include surgical excision, shave excision, laser therapy, and cryotherapy (freezing). The choice of treatment depends on factors such as the size, location, and type of mole.

Skin Cancer Surveillance: Individuals with a history of atypical or cancerous moles, as well as those with risk factors for melanoma, may require regular skin cancer screenings to monitor for new or changing moles and detect skin cancer at an early stage when it is most treatable.

❖ ❖ ❖ ❖

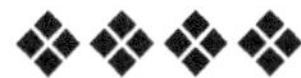

MORPHEA (त्वककाठिन्य)

Morphea According to Ayurveda

Morphea is a skin condition characterized by patches of hardened, discolored skin that typically appear on the abdomen, chest, or back. According to Ayurveda, Morphea is understood as a manifestation of an imbalance in the body's doshas, particularly Vata and Kapha.

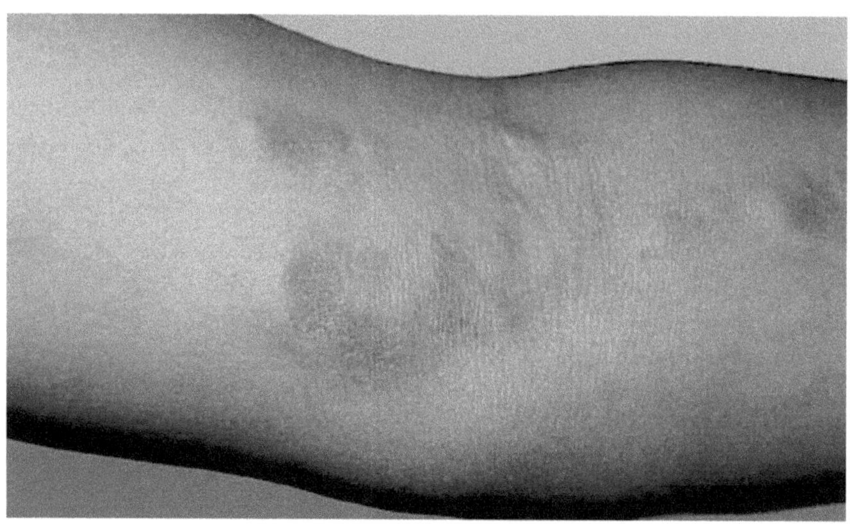

From an Ayurvedic perspective, Morphea is primarily associated with an imbalance in Vata dosha, which governs movement and circulation in the body. When Vata becomes aggravated, it can lead to dryness, roughness, and unevenness in the skin, which are characteristic features of Morphea.

Furthermore, Kapha dosha, which governs structure and lubrication in the body, may also play a role in Morphea. An excess of Kapha can lead to the accumulation of toxins in the body, which may manifest as skin abnormalities like Morphea.

Ayurvedic treatment for Morphea focuses on restoring balance to the doshas through a combination of dietary and lifestyle modifications, herbal remedies, and detoxification therapies. Here are some Ayurvedic approaches that may be used to address Morphea:

Dietary Modifications: A diet that pacifies Vata and Kapha doshas is typically recommended for individuals with Morphea. This includes consuming warm, cooked foods and avoiding cold, raw, and processed foods. Additionally, incorporating spices such as turmeric, ginger, and cumin can help reduce inflammation and promote skin health.

Herbal Remedies: Ayurvedic herbs known for their detoxifying and rejuvenating properties may be prescribed to cleanse the body of accumulated toxins and support skin health. Some commonly used herbs for Morphea include neem, turmeric, manjistha, and guggul.

External Therapies: External applications of herbal oils and pastes may be used to nourish and moisturize the skin, reduce inflammation, and promote healing. Herbal oils such as sesame oil or coconut oil infused with anti-inflammatory herbs can be massaged onto the affected areas to improve circulation and alleviate dryness.

Detoxification Therapies: Panchakarma, which is a comprehensive Ayurvedic detoxification therapy, may be recommended to remove toxins from the body and restore balance to the doshas. This may involve procedures such as Abhyanga (therapeutic oil massage), Swedana (herbal steam therapy), and Basti (medicated enema therapy).

Stress Management: Stress can exacerbate imbalances in the doshas and worsen skin conditions like Morphea. Practices such as yoga, meditation, and pranayama (breathing exercises) can help reduce stress levels and promote overall well-being.

It's important to note that Ayurvedic treatment should be personalized based on an individual's unique constitution (prakriti) and the underlying cause of Morphea. Consulting with a qualified Ayurvedic practitioner can help determine the most appropriate treatment plan for addressing Morphea and restoring balance to the body. Additionally, it's advisable to seek medical advice and combine Ayurvedic treatment with conventional medical care for comprehensive management of Morphea.

Morphea in Modern Medicine

In modern medicine, Morphea, also known as localized scleroderma, is considered an autoimmune condition that affects the skin and sometimes underlying tissues. While the exact cause of Morphea is not fully understood, it is believed to involve an abnormal immune response leading to inflammation and excessive collagen production in the affected areas.

Morphea is a relatively rare autoimmune disorder characterized by localized patches of thickened, hardened, and discolored skin. It primarily affects the skin but can also involve underlying tissues such as fat, muscle, and bone. Morphea is classified into several subtypes based on the extent and distribution of skin involvement, with the most common form being plaque morphea, characterized by oval-shaped or linear patches of hardened skin.

The exact cause of Morphea is not fully understood, but it is thought to result from an abnormal immune response leading to inflammation and excessive collagen deposition in the affected areas. Genetic factors, environmental triggers, and abnormalities in the immune system are believed to contribute to the development of Morphea. However, the specific triggers and mechanisms vary from person to person.

Morphea typically presents with one or more localized patches of hardened skin, which may be white, yellowish, or reddish in color. The skin lesions are usually firm to the touch and may be surrounded by a lighter or darker border. In some cases, Morphea can cause itching, pain, or restriction of movement if the lesions affect underlying tissues.

Diagnosis of Morphea is based on clinical evaluation, including a thorough medical history and physical examination. In some cases, additional tests such as skin biopsy, imaging studies, or blood tests may be performed to rule out other conditions and assess the extent of involvement.

Treatment for Morphea aims to control symptoms, minimize disease activity, and prevent complications. The approach to treatment may vary depending on the severity and extent of skin involvement, as well as individual factors such as age, overall health, and treatment goals. Common treatment options for Morphea include:

Topical Therapies: Topical medications such as corticosteroids, calcineurin inhibitors, or vitamin D analogs may be applied directly to the skin lesions to reduce inflammation and soften the hardened skin.

Phototherapy: Phototherapy, including ultraviolet A (UVA) or ultraviolet B (UVB) light therapy, may be used to treat Morphea by suppressing inflammation and promoting skin healing. Phototherapy is often combined with psoralen, a light-sensitizing medication, to enhance its effectiveness.

Systemic Therapies: In cases of more widespread or severe Morphea, oral medications such as corticosteroids, methotrexate, mycophenolate mofetil, or hydroxychloroquine may be prescribed to suppress the immune system and reduce inflammation.

Physical Therapy: Physical therapy techniques such as stretching exercises, massage, and joint mobilization may be recommended to improve flexibility, reduce pain, and prevent joint stiffness in individuals with Morphea affecting underlying tissues.

Surgery: In rare cases, surgical procedures such as fat grafting or tissue expansion may be considered to correct deformities or restore function in severely affected areas of the body.

It's important for individuals with Morphea to work closely with healthcare providers, including dermatologists and rheumatologists, to develop a personalized treatment plan tailored to their specific needs and preferences. Regular monitoring and follow-up evaluations are essential to assess treatment response, manage potential side effects, and adjust treatment as needed to optimize outcomes.

While Morphea is generally considered a chronic condition, many people experience periods of remission or stabilization with appropriate treatment. However, Morphea can have a significant impact on quality of life due to its physical and psychological effects, including changes in appearance, functional limitations, and emotional distress. Supportive care, patient education, and psychosocial interventions may be helpful in addressing these aspects of Morphea management and promoting overall well-being.

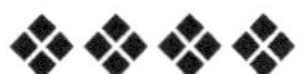

ONYCHOMYCOSIS (नखकवकता)

Onychomycosis According to Ayurveda

Onychomycosis, commonly known as nail fungus, is a fungal infection of the nails that affects millions of people worldwide. In Ayurveda, this condition is referred to as **"Nakha Kawakta"** Ayurveda, the ancient Indian system of medicine, offers a holistic approach to health and wellness, addressing the root cause of diseases rather than just the symptoms.

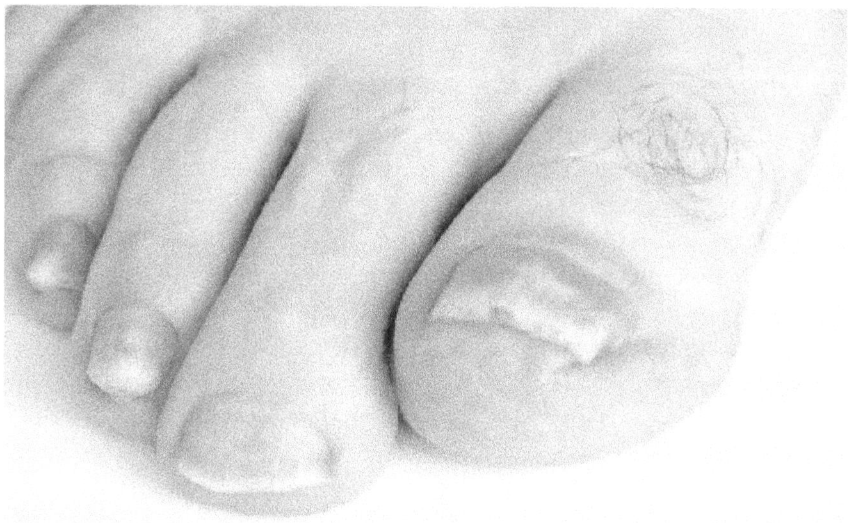

Causes According to Ayurveda: In Ayurveda, onychomycosis is believed to be caused by an imbalance of the Pitta and Kapha doshas, which govern various physiological functions in the body. Excessive consumption of Pitta-aggravating foods such as spicy, oily, and acidic foods, as well as Kapha-aggravating foods such as dairy products and sweets, can disrupt the balance of these doshas, leading to the development of fungal infections like onychomycosis.

Symptoms According to Ayurveda: Ayurveda identifies several symptoms associated with onychomycosis, including:

Discoloration of the nails, ranging from yellowish-brown to black.

Thickening of the nails, making them appear distorted and brittle.
Crumbling or flaking of the nails.
Itching and irritation around the affected nails.
Foul odor emanating from the infected nails.

Ayurvedic Treatment Approaches: Ayurvedic treatment for onychomycosis aims to rebalance the doshas, strengthen the immune system, and eliminate the fungal infection. Treatment modalities may include:

Dietary Modifications: Following a Pitta and Kapha pacifying diet, avoiding spicy, oily, and acidic foods, and incorporating cooling and detoxifying foods such as fresh fruits, vegetables, and herbs.

Herbal Remedies: Ayurvedic herbs with antifungal properties, such as neem (Azadirachta indica), turmeric (Curcuma longa), and garlic (Allium sativum), may be used internally and externally to combat the fungal infection.

Detoxification Therapies: Panchakarma therapies, including Virechana (therapeutic purgation) and Raktamokshana (bloodletting), may be recommended to eliminate toxins from the body and purify the blood.

External Treatments: Topical applications of herbal pastes, oils, or powders containing antifungal ingredients may be used to treat the infected nails and surrounding skin.

Lifestyle Recommendations: Adopting a healthy lifestyle, practicing good nail hygiene, wearing breathable footwear, and maintaining proper foot hygiene can help prevent the recurrence of onychomycosis.

Onychomycosis in Modern Medicine

Onychomycosis, also known as nail fungus, is a common fungal infection affecting the nails, primarily the toenails. In modern medicine, onychomycosis is recognized as a dermatophytic infection caused by various fungi, including dermatophytes, yeasts, and molds. Here's an essay detailing onychomycosis in modern medicine:

Onychomycosis is a prevalent fungal infection of the nails, characterized by discoloration, thickening, and deformity of the nails. It can lead to cosmetic concerns as well as discomfort and pain in severe cases. Modern medicine recognizes several types of onychomycosis, including distal subungual onychomycosis, proximal subungual onychomycosis, and superficial white onychomycosis, each caused by different fungal organisms.

Causes and Risk Factors: Onychomycosis is primarily caused by dermatophytes, fungi that thrive in warm, moist environments such as shoes and socks. Other fungi such as yeasts and molds can also cause nail infections. Risk factors for developing onychomycosis include advanced age, diabetes, peripheral vascular disease, immunodeficiency, trauma to the nails, and frequent exposure to moisture.

Symptoms and Diagnosis: Symptoms of onychomycosis include nail discoloration (yellow, brown, or black), thickening of the nails, crumbling or brittleness, distorted nail shape, and separation of the nail from the nail bed. Diagnosis is typically made through clinical examination, nail sampling for laboratory analysis (potassium hydroxide preparation, fungal culture), and sometimes, biopsy for histopathological examination.

Treatment Approaches: Modern medicine offers various treatment options for onychomycosis, including topical antifungal medications, oral antifungal drugs, and in some cases, surgical intervention (nail avulsion). Oral antifungal agents such as terbinafine and itraconazole are often considered the first-line treatment for moderate to severe cases of onychomycosis, with topical antifungals being used for milder infections. However, these treatments may have side effects and require prolonged therapy.

Prevention Strategies: Preventing onychomycosis involves practicing good foot hygiene, keeping nails clean and trimmed, wearing breathable footwear, avoiding walking barefoot in public areas such as pools and locker rooms, and treating fungal skin infections promptly. Additionally, individuals with risk factors for onychomycosis should be vigilant about nail care and seek medical attention if they suspect an infection.

Paronychia According to Ayurveda

Paronychia, known as "Nakhapaka" in Ayurveda, is a condition affecting the nails and surrounding tissues, characterized by inflammation and infection. In Ayurveda, Paronychia is primarily attributed to an imbalance in the "Vata" and "Kapha" doshas, which are the fundamental energies governing the body. When these doshas are aggravated, they can lead to various disorders, including Paronychia.

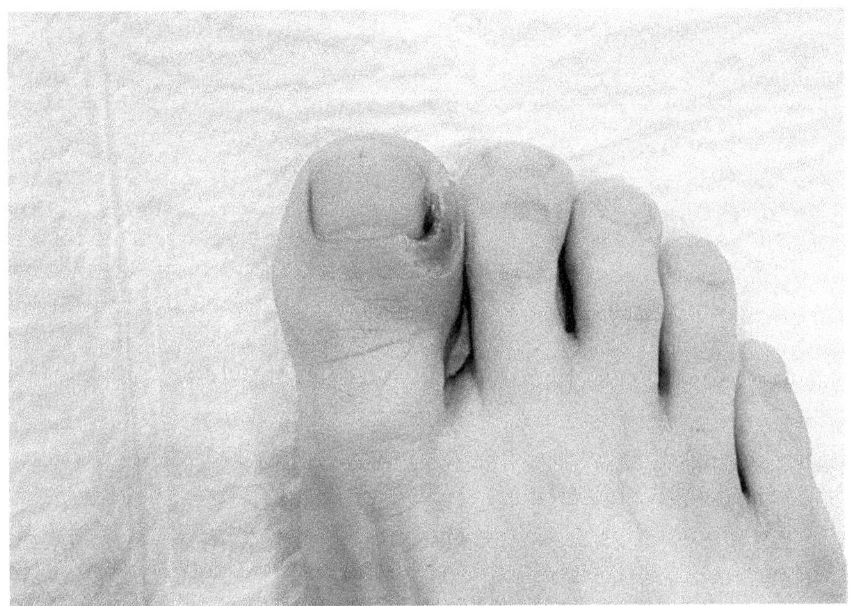

According to Ayurvedic Principles, Paronychia Can Manifest Due To Several Factors:

Dietary Factors: Consumption of excessive dry, spicy, and cold foods can aggravate Vata and Kapha doshas, contributing to Paronychia. Additionally, the ingestion of incompatible foods (viruddha ahara) or foods causing ama (toxins) formation may also play a role.

Poor Hygiene: Improper nail care, such as cutting nails too short or biting them, can create openings for pathogens to enter, leading to infection and inflammation around the nails.

Trauma: Physical injury or trauma to the nails or surrounding tissues can disrupt the natural balance of doshas, predisposing one to Paronychia.

Weak Immune System: A compromised immune system due to factors such as stress, fatigue, or underlying health conditions can increase susceptibility to Paronychia.

Ayurvedic management of Paronychia involves a combination of dietary and lifestyle modifications, herbal remedies, and external therapies tailored to address the underlying imbalances. Here is a detailed approach to managing Paronychia in Ayurveda:

Dietary Recommendations: Emphasize warm, nourishing foods that pacify Vata and Kapha doshas, such as cooked vegetables, whole grains, soups, and herbal teas.
Avoid cold, dry, and spicy foods, as well as foods that are difficult to digest.
Stay hydrated by consuming warm water throughout the day to help flush out toxins from the body.

Lifestyle Modifications: Maintain proper nail hygiene by keeping nails clean and trimmed, avoiding excessive cutting or biting.
Practice stress-reducing techniques such as yoga, meditation, and deep breathing exercises to balance the nervous system and strengthen immunity.
Ensure an adequate amount of sleep and rest to support the body's natural healing processes.

Herbal Remedies: Internal herbal preparations may include formulations containing herbs like neem (Azadirachta indica), turmeric (Curcuma longa), and guggulu (Commiphora wightii) to purify the blood, reduce inflammation, and strengthen immunity.

External applications of herbal pastes or oils containing ingredients like turmeric, neem, and manjistha (Rubia cordifolia) can help reduce swelling, pain, and infection around the affected nails.

External Therapies: Warm oil massages, especially with sesame or coconut oil infused with anti-inflammatory herbs, can promote circulation and aid in the healing process.

Steam therapy (swedana) using medicated herbs can help alleviate pain, reduce inflammation, and detoxify the affected area.

Panchakarma Detoxification: In severe or chronic cases, undergoing Panchakarma therapies like Virechana (therapeutic purgation) or Rakta Mokshana (bloodletting) under the supervision of a qualified Ayurvedic practitioner may be beneficial to eliminate toxins and restore doshic balance.

Paronychia in Modern Medicine

In modern medicine, Paronychia is defined as an infection of the skin around the fingernails or toenails, typically caused by bacteria or fungi. There are two main types of Paronychia: acute and chronic.

Acute Paronychia: This type usually develops over a few hours or days and is often caused by bacterial infections, most commonly Staphylococcus aureus. Factors such as nail biting, finger sucking, manicures, or injuries to the nail fold can predispose individuals to acute Paronychia. The infection typically presents with pain, redness, swelling, and pus formation around the nail.

Chronic Paronychia: Chronic Paronychia develops gradually over weeks or months and is more commonly associated with fungal infections, particularly Candida species. It is often seen in individuals whose hands are frequently exposed to moisture, such as dishwashers, bartenders, or healthcare workers. Chronic Paronychia may also result from repeated exposure to irritants or allergens.

Diagnosis and Treatment:

Diagnosis of Paronychia is primarily clinical, based on the characteristic symptoms and physical examination findings. In some cases, laboratory tests such as bacterial or fungal cultures may be performed to identify the causative organism.

Treatment of Paronychia typically involves conservative measures for acute cases, including warm water soaks, proper nail hygiene, and topical or oral antibiotics in bacterial infections. For chronic Paronychia, antifungal medications may be prescribed, along with measures to keep the affected area dry and clean.

In severe or recurrent cases, surgical intervention may be necessary to drain abscesses or remove damaged tissue around the nail fold.

Preventive Measures: Maintaining good nail hygiene, including regular trimming and avoiding trauma to the nail fold, can help prevent Paronychia.

Individuals at risk, such as healthcare workers or those with frequent exposure to moisture, should wear gloves to protect their hands and nails.

Avoiding nail biting, finger sucking, or aggressive manicuring can also reduce the risk of developing Paronychia.

Complications: If left untreated or if the infection spreads, Paronychia can lead to complications such as cellulitis (infection of deeper tissues), abscess formation, or even systemic infection in severe cases.

Chronic Paronychia may result in nail deformities or permanent damage to the nail bed if not properly managed

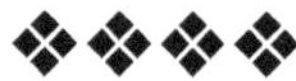

PEDICULOSIS (जुएं)

Pediculosis According to Ayurveda

Pediculosis, commonly known as "lice infestation," is a parasitic condition caused by the presence of lice on the human body. In Ayurveda, pediculosis is referred to as "Sarameeha" or "Kutaja," and it is classified under the category of "Kshudra rogas" (minor diseases).

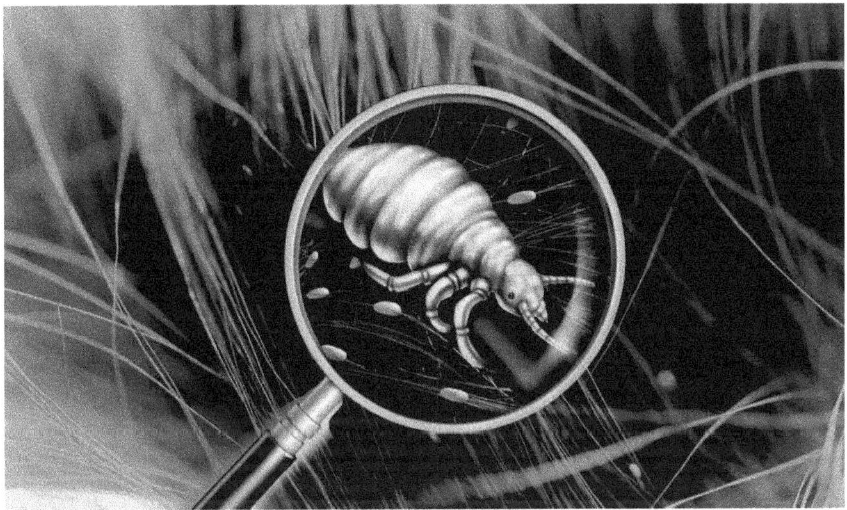

According to Ayurveda, pediculosis is primarily caused by an imbalance in the "Kapha" and "Pitta" doshas. Excessive intake of sweet, oily, and cold foods can aggravate Kapha dosha, leading to conditions favorable for lice infestation. Additionally, excessive heat in the body, resulting from an aggravated Pitta dosha, can also contribute to pediculosis.

Ayurvedic treatment for pediculosis involves a combination of internal medication, external applications, and lifestyle modifications.

Internal Medication: Ayurvedic practitioners may prescribe herbal formulations to balance the doshas and strengthen the immune system. These formulations may include herbs like neem (Azadirachta indica), turmeric (Curcuma longa), and triphala (a combination of three fruits: Amalaki, Bibhitaki, and Haritaki) to purify the blood and detoxify the body.

External Applications: Herbal oils and pastes are commonly used externally to eliminate lice and soothe the scalp. Neem oil, coconut oil infused with neem leaves, or a paste made from neem leaves and turmeric can be applied to the scalp and hair. These natural remedies not only kill lice but also help in relieving itching and inflammation.

Personal Hygiene: Maintaining personal hygiene is crucial in preventing and managing pediculosis. Regular washing of hair with herbal shampoos, combing with a fine-toothed comb to remove lice and nits (lice eggs), and avoiding sharing personal items such as combs, hats, and towels can prevent the spread of lice infestation.

Dietary Recommendations: Ayurveda emphasizes dietary modifications to balance the doshas. Individuals with pediculosis are advised to avoid excessive consumption of sweet, oily, and cold foods, as these can aggravate Kapha dosha. Instead, a diet rich in bitter, pungent, and astringent tastes is recommended to pacify Kapha and Pitta doshas.

Lifestyle Modifications: Stress and lack of sleep can weaken the immune system, making the body more susceptible to infections, including pediculosis. Practicing stress-relief techniques such as yoga, meditation, and adequate sleep can support overall health and enhance the body's natural defenses against lice infestation.

Pediculosis in Modern Medicine

In modern medicine, pediculosis, commonly referred to as lice infestation, is recognized as a contagious parasitic condition caused by the presence of lice on the human body. There are three main types of lice that infest humans: head lice (Pediculus humanus capitis), body lice (Pediculus humanus corporis), and pubic lice (Pthirus pubis).

Causes and Transmission: Lice infestations occur when lice crawl onto the skin or hair and feed on blood. Transmission commonly occurs through direct contact with infected individuals or through sharing personal items such as combs, brushes, hats, and clothing. Poor personal hygiene and overcrowded living conditions can also contribute to the spread of lice infestations.

Symptoms: The main symptom of pediculosis is itching, which is caused by the body's allergic reaction to lice bites. Scratching the affected areas can lead to secondary bacterial infections. Other symptoms may include the presence of lice or their eggs (nits) on the scalp, body, or pubic region, as well as irritability and difficulty sleeping due to itching.

Diagnosis: Diagnosis of pediculosis is typically based on the identification of live lice or nits in the hair or on the body. Fine-toothed combs, known as nit combs, may be used to comb through the hair and detect lice and nits. Additionally, skin scrapings or adhesive tape tests may be performed to collect samples for microscopic examination.

Treatment: The primary goal of treatment is to eliminate lice and their eggs while minimizing skin irritation and preventing reinfestation. Over-the-counter (OTC) and prescription medications, such as pyrethrin or permethrin-based shampoos and lotions, are commonly used to kill lice. In cases of treatment-resistant lice, oral medications or alternative treatments, such as dimethicone-based products or manual removal, may be recommended.

Prevention: Prevention strategies include practicing good personal hygiene, avoiding close contact with infected individuals, and refraining from sharing personal items. Regular washing of clothing, bedding, and other potentially contaminated items in hot water and drying them on high heat can help kill lice and prevent reinfestation.

Public Health Concerns: Although pediculosis is not considered a serious medical condition, it can cause significant discomfort and social stigma. In certain settings, such as schools, childcare facilities, and homeless shelters, outbreaks of lice infestations can occur, leading to public health concerns and the need for prompt treatment and preventive measures.

Pellegra According to Ayurveda

In Ayurveda, Pellegra is a condition characterized by a set of symptoms primarily affecting the skin, digestive system, and nervous system. Pellegra corresponds closely to the Western medical condition of pellagra, which is caused by a deficiency of niacin (vitamin B3), leading to a triad of symptoms: dermatitis, diarrhea, and dementia.

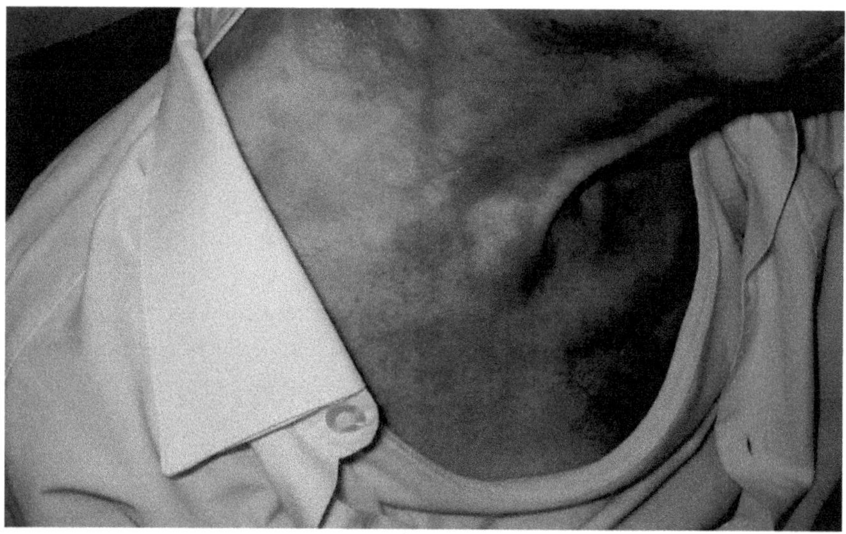

In Ayurveda, Pellegra is understood through the lens of doshas (biological energies), dhatus (tissues), and malas (waste products). According to Ayurvedic principles, an imbalance in the doshas, particularly pitta and vata, along with impaired agni (digestive fire) and accumulation of ama (toxins), contributes to the manifestation of Pellegra.

Etiology (Nidana):

Dietary Factors: A diet deficient in niacin-rich foods such as whole grains, legumes, nuts, and meat can lead to a deficiency of this vital nutrient, contributing to the onset of Pellegra.

Impaired Digestion (Mandagni): Weak digestive fire compromises the proper metabolism and assimilation of nutrients, including niacin, leading to its deficiency in the body.

Dosha Imbalance: An aggravated pitta dosha coupled with vata vitiation plays a significant role in the pathogenesis of Pellegra. Pitta, when aggravated, can impair the skin and digestive system, while vata exacerbation contributes to neurological manifestations.

Toxic Buildup (Ama): Poor digestion results in the accumulation of ama, or metabolic toxins, which further obstructs the channels of the body and hampers the proper functioning of tissues and organs.

Clinical Features (Lakshanas):

Skin Manifestations: The skin is often the first to show signs of Pellegra, presenting with a characteristic dermatitis marked by erythema, scaling, and hyperpigmentation. The affected areas may exhibit a rough, scaly texture resembling a sunburn, especially in sun-exposed areas.

Gastrointestinal Symptoms: Digestive disturbances such as diarrhea, abdominal pain, nausea, and loss of appetite are common in Pellegra. The bowel movements may be frequent, loose, and accompanied by foul-smelling stools.

Neurological Symptoms: As the condition progresses, neurological symptoms become evident, including cognitive impairment, confusion, memory loss, insomnia, and peripheral neuropathy. Patients may experience weakness, tingling, and numbness in the extremities.

Ayurvedic Management (Chikitsa):

Dietary Modifications: Emphasize a balanced diet rich in niacin-containing foods such as whole grains, pulses, nuts, seeds, green leafy vegetables, and animal proteins. Avoid excessive consumption of refined carbohydrates, processed foods, and alcohol.

Herbal Remedies: Ayurvedic herbs like Brahmi (Bacopa monnieri), Ashwagandha (Withania somnifera), and Shatavari (Asparagus racemosus) can help improve cognitive function, reduce inflammation, and support nervous system health.

Panchakarma Therapies: Detoxification therapies such as Virechana (therapeutic purgation) and Basti (medicated enema) are beneficial for eliminating ama and restoring doshic balance.

Lifestyle Modifications: Encourage regular exercise, stress management techniques such as yoga and meditation, and adequate rest to support overall health and well-being.

Prognosis (Upashaya):

With early intervention and appropriate treatment, the prognosis for Pellegra in Ayurveda is generally favorable. Symptomatic relief can be achieved, and the progression of the disease can be halted or reversed with holistic management approaches focusing on addressing the underlying imbalances.

Pellegra in Modern Medicine

In modern medicine, Pellegra, also known as pellagra, is a nutritional deficiency disorder caused by a deficiency of niacin (vitamin B3) and/or tryptophan, an essential amino acid that serves as a precursor to niacin. Here's an essay on Pellegra in modern medicine:

Pellagra is a nutritional deficiency disorder characterized by a deficiency of niacin (vitamin B3) and/or tryptophan, leading to a spectrum of symptoms affecting the skin, digestive system, and nervous system. The condition was first described in the early 20th century, primarily in populations subsisting on diets lacking in niacin-rich foods.

Etiology:

Dietary Insufficiency: Pellagra typically arises in individuals with diets deficient in niacin-containing foods such as meat, fish, poultry, legumes, nuts, and whole grains. Consumption of predominantly maize-based diets, which are low in bioavailable niacin and contain niacin-binding substances, predisposes individuals to pellagra.

Impaired Tryptophan Conversion: In addition to dietary insufficiency, impaired conversion of tryptophan to niacin due to factors such as gastrointestinal disorders or medications can contribute to the development of pellagra.

Clinical Features:

Dermatological Manifestations: Pellagra classically presents with a triad of dermatitis characterized by symmetric erythema, scaling, and hyperpigmentation, particularly in sun-exposed areas. The skin lesions may progress to vesicular and bullous eruptions, leading to ulceration and scarring if left untreated.

Gastrointestinal Symptoms: Patients with pellagra often experience gastrointestinal disturbances such as diarrhea, abdominal pain, nausea, vomiting, and anorexia. The diarrhea is typically watery and malodorous, resembling a "rice-water" stool.

Neurological Symptoms: Neurological manifestations of pellagra include cognitive impairment, confusion, memory loss, insomnia, anxiety, depression, peripheral neuropathy, and hallucinations. Severe cases may progress to delirium, seizures, and coma.

Diagnostic Evaluation:

Clinical Assessment: Diagnosis of pellagra is primarily based on clinical features, including the characteristic dermatitis, gastrointestinal symptoms, and neurological manifestations. A thorough dietary history and physical examination are essential for identifying risk factors and assessing symptom severity.

Laboratory Testing: Laboratory investigations may reveal decreased levels of serum niacin and tryptophan, along with alterations in biochemical markers such as reduced urinary excretion of metabolites associated with niacin metabolism.

Treatment And Prevention:

Niacin Supplementation: Treatment of pellagra involves oral or parenteral supplementation with niacin (nicotinic acid or nicotinamide) to correct the deficiency and alleviate symptoms. Dosage and route of administration depend on the severity of the condition and individual patient factors.

Dietary Modification: Emphasizing a balanced diet rich in niacin-containing foods and protein sources is essential for preventing pellagra. Fortification of staple foods with niacin and educational interventions aimed at improving dietary diversity can help reduce the incidence of pellagra in at-risk populations.

Prognosis:

With prompt diagnosis and appropriate treatment, the prognosis for pellagra is favorable, and symptom resolution can be achieved within weeks of niacin supplementation. However, untreated or severe cases may result in irreversible complications and increased morbidity and mortality.

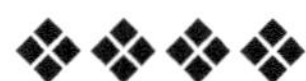

PEMPHIGUS (पेम्फीगस)

Pemphigus According to Ayurveda

Pemphigus, known as "पेम्फीगस" in Ayurveda, is a rare autoimmune disease characterized by the formation of blisters on the skin and mucous membranes.

Ayurveda views pemphigus as a manifestation of underlying imbalances in the body's dhatus (tissues) and doshas (energies). The accumulation of ama (toxins) due to impaired digestion and metabolism is believed to play a significant role in the development of pemphigus.

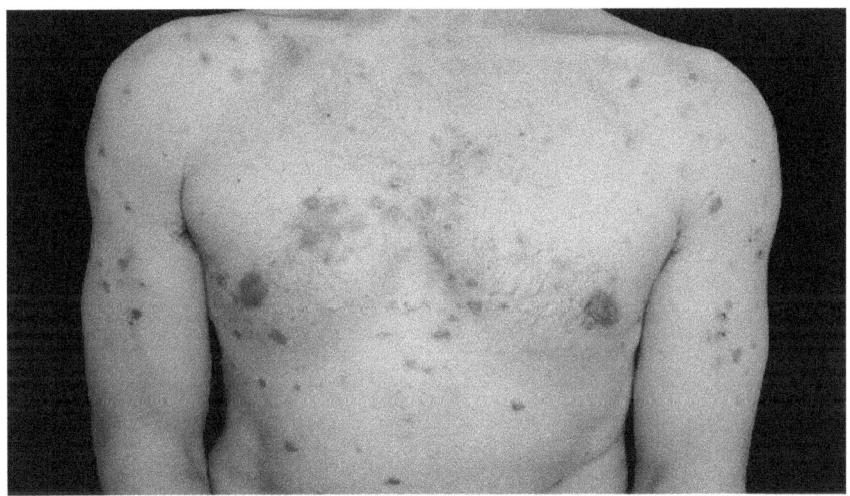

According To Ayurvedic Principles, The Following Factors Can Contribute To The Development Of Pemphigus:

Aggravation of Pitta Dosha: Pitta dosha governs the metabolic processes in the body. When Pitta becomes aggravated due to factors such as excessive consumption of spicy, sour, and salty foods, exposure to excessive heat, and emotional stress, it can lead to inflammation and disruption of the body's natural healing mechanisms.

Imbalance in Kapha Dosha: Kapha dosha governs the structure and lubrication of the body. When Kapha becomes imbalanced due to factors such as consuming heavy and oily foods, lack of exercise, and sedentary lifestyle, it can lead to the accumulation of ama (toxins) in the body, further exacerbating the symptoms of pemphigus.

Weak Digestive Fire (Agni): Ayurveda emphasizes the importance of a strong digestive fire (agni) for the proper digestion and metabolism of food. When agni is weak, it can lead to the accumulation of undigested food particles (ama) in the body, which can contribute to the development of skin diseases such as pemphigus.

Impaired Immune Function: Ayurveda recognizes the role of the immune system in protecting the body from disease. When the immune system becomes compromised due to factors such as poor diet, stress, and unhealthy lifestyle habits, it can lead to an increased susceptibility to autoimmune conditions like pemphigus.

Ayurvedic treatment for pemphigus aims to address the underlying imbalances in the body's doshas and promote overall health and well-being. Treatment modalities may include:

Dietary Modifications: Following a Pitta-pacifying diet that is cooling, soothing, and easy to digest can help alleviate symptoms of pemphigus. This may include incorporating foods such as fresh fruits, vegetables, whole grains, and cooling herbs like coriander, mint, and fennel into the diet while avoiding spicy, sour, and oily foods.

Herbal Remedies: Ayurvedic herbs such as neem (Azadirachta indica), turmeric (Curcuma longa), aloe vera (Aloe barbadensis), and guduchi (Tinospora cordifolia) are known for their anti-inflammatory, immunomodulatory, and detoxifying properties, which can help alleviate symptoms and promote healing in pemphigus.

Panchakarma Therapy: Panchakarma, a detoxification therapy in Ayurveda, may be recommended to eliminate ama (toxins) from the body and restore balance to the doshas. This may include procedures such as vamana (therapeutic vomiting), virechana (purgation), and basti (medicated enema), depending on the individual's constitution and condition.

Lifestyle Modifications: Adopting a healthy lifestyle that includes regular exercise, stress management techniques such as yoga and meditation, adequate rest, and maintaining proper hygiene can help support the body's natural healing process and prevent recurrence of symptoms.

Ayurvedic Medications: Ayurvedic formulations containing a combination of herbs and minerals tailored to individual needs may be prescribed to address specific symptoms and imbalances in pemphigus.

Pemphigus in Modern Medicine

In modern medicine, pemphigus is recognized as a rare autoimmune disorder characterized by the formation of blisters on the skin and mucous membranes. It is considered to be caused by an autoimmune reaction in which the body's immune system mistakenly attacks healthy cells in the skin and mucous membranes, leading to the formation of blisters and erosions.

The exact cause of pemphigus is not fully understood, but it is believed to involve a combination of genetic predisposition, environmental factors, and immune dysregulation. Factors such as certain medications, infections, and environmental triggers may also play a role in triggering or exacerbating the disease.

Pemphigus Can Be Classified Into Several Subtypes, Including:

Pemphigus Vulgaris: The most common form of pemphigus, characterized by painful blisters and erosions on the skin and mucous membranes.

Pemphigus Foliaceus: Characterized by superficial blisters and erosions primarily on the skin, often with less involvement of the mucous membranes.

Paraneoplastic Pemphigus: A rare subtype of pemphigus associated with underlying malignancies, often involving multiple organ systems and severe mucosal involvement.

Diagnosis of pemphigus typically involves a combination of clinical evaluation, skin biopsy, and immunological tests such as direct and indirect immunofluorescence microscopy to detect antibodies targeting components of the skin and mucous membranes.

Treatment of pemphigus in modern medicine usually involves a combination of immunosuppressive medications and supportive care to control symptoms, promote healing, and prevent complications. Commonly used medications may include corticosteroids, immunosuppressants such as azathioprine, mycophenolate mofetil, or rituximab, and adjuvant therapies such as topical treatments and wound care.

Management of pemphigus in modern medicine also involves close monitoring of disease activity, regular follow-up visits with healthcare providers, and collaboration with specialists such as dermatologists, immunologists, and rheumatologists to optimize treatment and minimize side effects.

In severe cases of pemphigus that are refractory to conventional treatments, other therapeutic options such as intravenous immunoglobulin therapy, plasmapheresis, or immunomodulatory agents may be considered.

Overall, while pemphigus remains a challenging condition to manage, advances in modern medicine have led to significant improvements in diagnosis, treatment, and outcomes for patients with this autoimmune disorder. However, ongoing research is needed to further understand the underlying mechanisms of pemphigus and develop more targeted and effective therapies.

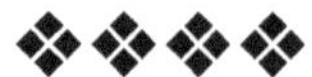

Prickly Heat According to Ayurveda

Prickly heat, known as "ghamoriya" in Ayurveda, is a common skin condition caused by excessive sweating during hot and humid weather

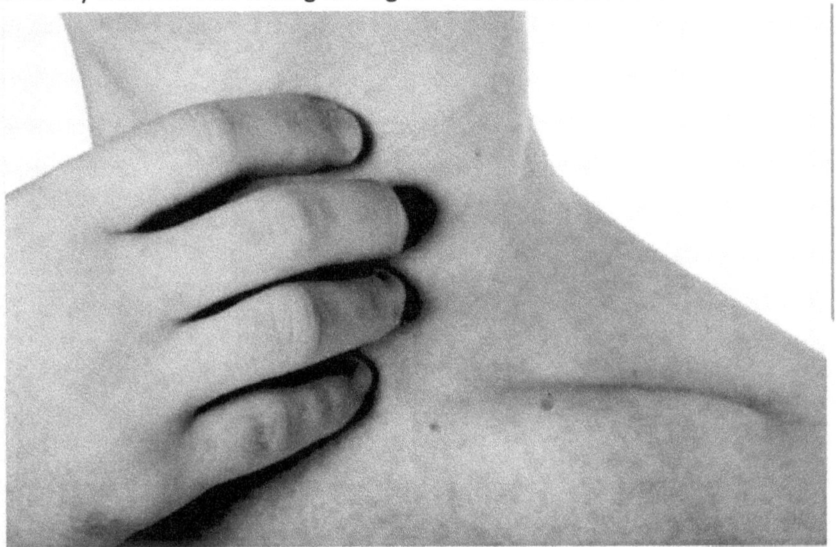

Causes According To Ayurveda: Ayurveda attributes the onset of prickly heat to an imbalance in the body's doshas, especially Pitta and Kapha. Pitta dosha governs metabolism, digestion, and body temperature regulation, while Kapha dosha relates to moisture balance and skin health. Excessive consumption of Pitta-aggravating foods like spicy, oily, and acidic substances, combined with Kapha-aggravating factors such as excessive sweating, can disturb the equilibrium of these doshas, leading to the manifestation of prickly heat.

Symptoms: Prickly heat typically presents as small red bumps or rashes accompanied by intense itching and a prickling sensation. The affected areas, commonly the neck, back, chest, and groin, may experience discomfort and inflammation due to blocked sweat glands. In severe cases, blisters and pustules may form, exacerbating the discomfort.

Ayurvedic Treatment and Remedies: Ayurvedic management of prickly heat focuses on pacifying Pitta and Kapha doshas while promoting skin healing and rejuvenation. Here are some effective Ayurvedic remedies and treatments:

Dietary Modifications: Avoiding Pitta-aggravating foods such as spicy, oily, and fried items, and incorporating cooling, hydrating foods like cucumber, watermelon, and coconut water can help balance the body's internal heat.

Herbal Remedies: Ayurvedic herbs like neem, sandalwood, aloe vera, and coriander possess cooling and anti-inflammatory properties that soothe irritated skin and reduce itching. Applying their extracts or pastes topically can provide relief from prickly heat.

Ayurvedic Medications: Internal administration of herbs like triphala, guduchi, and manjistha helps detoxify the body, purify the blood, and alleviate Pitta-Kapha imbalances, thus addressing the root cause of prickly heat.

External Applications: Herbal powders or pastes containing ingredients like neem, turmeric, and sandalwood can be applied to the affected areas to alleviate itching, reduce inflammation, and promote healing.

Hygiene Practices: Keeping the skin clean and dry, wearing loose, breathable clothing made of natural fibers, and avoiding excessive exposure to heat and humidity are essential to prevent exacerbation of prickly heat.

Prickly Heat in Modern Medicine

Prickly heat, known as "ghamoriya" in Hindi, is a common skin condition also recognized in modern medicine. It is medically termed as miliaria, and it occurs when sweat becomes trapped in the sweat ducts, leading to inflammation and irritation of the skin.

Prickly heat, or miliaria, is a dermatological condition characterized by small, itchy red bumps on the skin. It commonly occurs in hot and humid environments where sweat production is high, and sweat ducts become blocked. Understanding the pathophysiology and management of prickly heat is essential in modern medicine to provide effective treatment and prevention strategies.

Causes According to Modern Medicine: Prickly heat occurs when sweat ducts become blocked, preventing sweat from reaching the surface of the skin. This blockage can be caused by various factors, including:

Hot and humid weather conditions that increase sweat production.
Prolonged physical activity or exertion leading to excessive sweating.
Occlusive clothing or fabrics that trap sweat against the skin.
Certain medications or medical conditions that affect sweat production or skin integrity.

Symptoms: The hallmark symptom of prickly heat is the appearance of small red bumps on the skin, often accompanied by itching and a prickling or tingling sensation. These bumps may be more prominent in areas where sweat tends to accumulate, such as the neck, back, chest, and groin. In severe cases, the blocked sweat ducts can lead to the formation of blisters or pustules.

Modern Treatment and Management: The management of prickly heat in modern medicine focuses on relieving symptoms, preventing further blockage of sweat ducts, and promoting skin healing. Treatment options include:

Topical Treatments: Calamine lotion, hydrocortisone cream, or menthol-containing lotions can help soothe itching and reduce inflammation.

Cooling Measures: Taking cool showers, applying cold compresses, or using air conditioning can help alleviate discomfort and reduce sweating.

Avoidance of Triggers: Avoiding hot and humid environments, wearing loose, breathable clothing, and using non-comedogenic skincare products can help prevent the recurrence of prickly heat.

Medications: In severe cases, oral antibiotics or corticosteroids may be prescribed to reduce inflammation and prevent secondary infections.

Prevention Strategies: Preventing prickly heat involves adopting measures to reduce sweating and keep the skin cool and dry. This includes:

Avoiding Excessive Heat And Humidity

Wearing loose, breathable clothing made of natural fibers.
Using talcum powder or antiperspirants to absorb excess sweat.
Taking frequent breaks during physical activity to cool down and rehydrate.

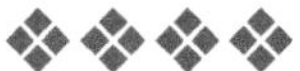

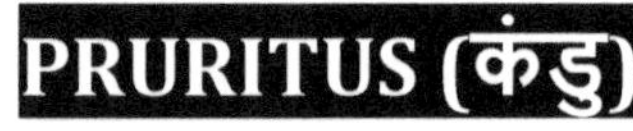

PRURITUS (कंडु)

Pruritus According to Ayurveda

Pruritus, commonly known as "कंडु" in Ayurveda, is a condition characterized by an itching sensation on the skin, often leading to scratching.

In Ayurveda, the skin is considered a reflection of the overall health of the body, and imbalances in the doshas can manifest as various skin disorders, including pruritus.

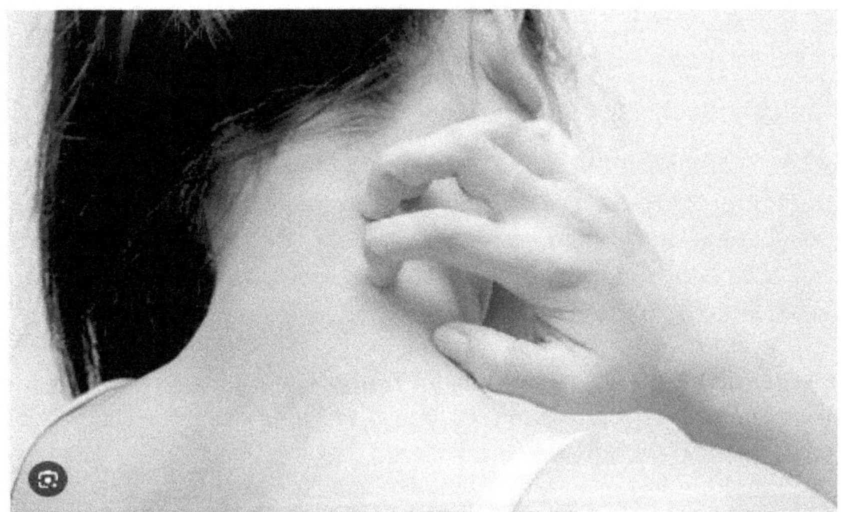

Pruritus, known as कंडु in Ayurveda, is a condition that affects the skin, leading to an intense itching sensation. It is a common complaint and can be caused by various factors, including imbalances in the doshas, poor diet, lifestyle factors, and environmental influences.

Etiology (Nidana): According to Ayurveda, pruritus can be caused by several factors:

Imbalance of Doshas: Pruritus is often associated with an imbalance in the Vata and Pitta doshas. Vata imbalance can lead to dryness and roughness of the skin, making it more prone to itching. Pitta imbalance can cause inflammation and heat in the body, aggravating the itching sensation.

Poor Diet: Consuming foods that are dry, spicy, and acidic can aggravate Pitta dosha, leading to pruritus. Additionally, consuming allergenic foods or foods that are difficult to digest can also contribute to the condition.

Environmental Factors: Exposure to harsh weather conditions, such as excessive heat or cold, can exacerbate pruritus. Dry and windy conditions can further aggravate Vata dosha, leading to dryness and itching of the skin.

Toxins (Ama): Accumulation of toxins in the body, known as Ama in Ayurveda, can impair the normal functioning of the skin and contribute to pruritus.

Symptoms (Lakshana): The primary symptom of pruritus is itching, which can range from mild to severe and may be accompanied by other symptoms such as redness, inflammation, and dryness of the skin. Scratching the affected area can lead to secondary complications such as skin lesions, infections, and scarring.

Treatment (Chikitsa): The treatment of pruritus in Ayurveda focuses on balancing the doshas, detoxifying the body, and nourishing the skin. Here are some common treatment approaches:

Dietary Modifications: Following a Pitta-pacifying diet, which includes cooling and hydrating foods such as fresh fruits, vegetables, and whole grains, can help alleviate pruritus. Avoiding spicy, oily, and processed foods is also recommended.

Herbal Remedies: Various herbs with cooling and anti-inflammatory properties can be used to alleviate itching and inflammation. Some commonly used herbs include neem, turmeric, aloe vera, and licorice.

Internal Cleansing (Panchakarma): Panchakarma therapies such as Virechana (therapeutic purgation) and Basti (medicated enema) can help remove toxins from the body and restore balance to the doshas.

External Therapies: External application of herbal oils and pastes can help soothe the skin and reduce itching. Herbal oils such as coconut oil, neem oil, and sesame oil are commonly used for this purpose.

Lifestyle Modifications: Avoiding exposure to harsh environmental conditions, practicing good hygiene, and managing stress through techniques such as yoga and meditation can also help prevent and alleviate pruritus.

Pruritus in Modern Medicine

In modern medicine, pruritus refers to the medical term for itching. It can occur due to various underlying conditions and is often considered a symptom rather than a standalone disease. Pruritus can affect any part of the body and may be acute or chronic in nature. Here's a detailed essay on pruritus in modern medicine:

Pruritus, commonly known as itching, is a sensation that prompts the desire to scratch the affected area. It is a common symptom experienced by people of all ages and can be caused by numerous factors, including skin conditions, systemic diseases, medications, and psychological factors.

Causes:

Skin Conditions: Pruritus can result from various skin conditions such as eczema, psoriasis, dermatitis, fungal infections, and dry skin. These conditions can disrupt the skin barrier, leading to irritation and itching.

Systemic Diseases: Certain systemic diseases such as liver disease (cholestasis), kidney disease (uremia), thyroid disorders, diabetes, and blood disorders can cause pruritus. These conditions may lead to biochemical changes in the body that contribute to itching.

Medications: Some medications, particularly those that affect the liver or kidney function, can cause pruritus as a side effect. Examples include opioid pain medications, certain antibiotics, antifungal drugs, and chemotherapy drugs.

Neurological Disorders: Neurological conditions such as multiple sclerosis, neuropathy, and pinched nerves can cause abnormal sensations, including itching, due to dysfunction of the nervous system.

Psychological Factors: Stress, anxiety, and depression can exacerbate itching sensations and lead to a cycle of itching and scratching, known as "itch-scratch cycle."

Diagnosis: Diagnosing the underlying cause of pruritus involves a thorough medical history, physical examination, and sometimes laboratory tests or imaging studies. The healthcare provider may inquire about the onset, duration, and characteristics of the itching, as well as any associated symptoms or triggers.

Treatment: The treatment of pruritus depends on identifying and addressing the underlying cause. Treatment approaches may include:

Topical Treatments: Topical corticosteroids, moisturizers, and antihistamine creams can help relieve itching associated with various skin conditions.

Oral Medications: Oral antihistamines, corticosteroids, and medications that target specific underlying conditions (e.g., liver disease, kidney disease) may be prescribed to alleviate itching.

Management of Underlying Conditions: Treating underlying systemic diseases or discontinuing medications that because itching can help alleviate pruritus.

Phototherapy: In some cases, phototherapy (light therapy) may be recommended to reduce inflammation and itching associated with certain skin conditions.

Behavioral Therapy: Cognitive-behavioral therapy (CBT) and relaxation techniques may be helpful in managing itching associated with psychological factors.

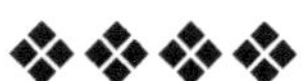

PSORIASIS (किटिभ)

Psoriasis According to Ayurveda

Psoriasis, known as "किटिभ" in Ayurveda, is a chronic autoimmune condition affecting the skin. According to Ayurveda, psoriasis is classified under "Kushtha" (skin disorders), specifically "Eka Kushtha" (a type of skin disorder involving vitiation of all three doshas - Vata, Pitta, and Kapha).

Ayurveda views psoriasis as a manifestation of an imbalance in the body's doshas, particularly Pitta and Kapha. It is believed that the accumulation of toxins (ama) in the body, improper diet and lifestyle, stress, and genetic predisposition contribute to the development of psoriasis.

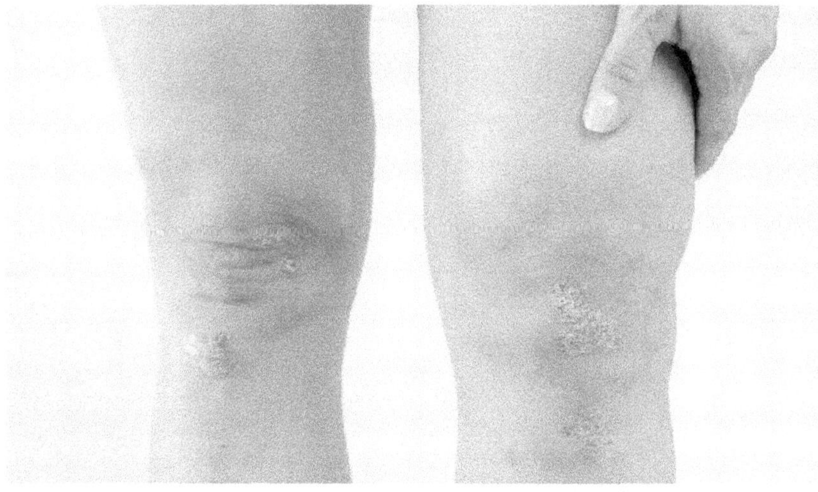

In Ayurveda, the treatment approach for psoriasis involves balancing the doshas, eliminating toxins from the body, and restoring skin health. Here are some key aspects of Ayurvedic management for psoriasis:

Purification Therapies (Panchakarma): Panchakarma procedures such as Vamana (therapeutic vomiting), Virechana (purgation), and Basti (medicated enema) are used to eliminate toxins from the body and balance the doshas. These therapies help in cleansing the body internally and promoting overall well-being.

Dietary Modifications: Ayurveda emphasizes the importance of following a Pitta and Kapha pacifying diet to alleviate symptoms of psoriasis. This includes consuming fresh fruits, vegetables, whole grains, and avoiding spicy, oily, and processed foods. Bitter and astringent tastes are preferred as they help in detoxifying the body.

Herbal Remedies: Various herbs are used in Ayurveda to manage psoriasis symptoms. Some commonly used herbs include Neem (Azadirachta indica), Turmeric (Curcuma longa), Aloe Vera (Aloe barbadensis), Manjistha (Rubia cordifolia), and Guduchi (Tinospora cordifolia). These herbs possess anti-inflammatory, detoxifying, and immune-modulating properties, which help in reducing skin inflammation and promoting healing.

External Therapies: External application of medicated oils, ointments, and pastes is an integral part of Ayurvedic treatment for psoriasis. Herbal oils such as Mahatiktaka Ghrita, Panchatikta Ghrita, and Nimba Taila are used for topical application to soothe the skin, reduce itching, and promote healing. Additionally, medicated baths (Sarvangadhara) and local fomentation (Pinda Sweda) with herbal decoctions are also beneficial.

Lifestyle Modifications: Ayurveda emphasizes the importance of maintaining a healthy lifestyle to manage psoriasis. Stress management techniques such as yoga, meditation, and pranayama (breathing exercises) are recommended to reduce stress levels, as stress can exacerbate psoriasis symptoms. Adequate sleep, regular exercise, and avoiding exposure to extreme weather conditions are also important.

Follow-Up Care: Ayurvedic treatment for psoriasis requires regular follow-up and monitoring to assess the progress of the condition. Adjustments to the treatment plan may be made based on the individual's response to therapy and changes in symptoms.

Psoriasis in Modern Medicine

Psoriasis is a chronic autoimmune disorder characterized by the rapid buildup of skin cells, resulting in thick, red patches with silvery scales on the skin's surface. In modern medicine, psoriasis is considered a multifactorial condition influenced by genetic predisposition, immune system dysfunction, environmental factors, and lifestyle choices.

Immune System Dysfunction: Psoriasis is primarily considered an immune-mediated disorder, involving abnormal activation of T cells in the immune system. In individuals with psoriasis, T cells mistakenly attack healthy skin cells, triggering inflammation and the rapid turnover of skin cells.

Genetic Predisposition: Family history plays a significant role in the development of psoriasis, with around one-third of patients having a family member with the condition. Multiple genes associated with immune system function, skin cell turnover, and inflammation have been identified as contributing factors to psoriasis susceptibility.

Environmental Triggers: Various environmental factors can exacerbate or trigger psoriasis flare-ups, including stress, infections (such as streptococcal throat infections), certain medications (such as lithium, beta-blockers, and antimalarial drugs), injury to the skin (such as cuts, burns, or insect bites), smoking, and excessive alcohol consumption.

Skin Cell Turnover: In individuals with psoriasis, the skin cell turnover process is significantly accelerated, leading to the rapid proliferation of keratinocytes (skin cells) and the formation of thickened patches of skin. This abnormal skin cell turnover results in the characteristic scaling and inflammation seen in psoriatic lesions.

Inflammatory Pathways: Psoriasis is associated with increased levels of pro-inflammatory cytokines, such as tumor necrosis factor-alpha (TNF-alpha), interleukin-17 (IL-17), and interleukin-23 (IL-23), which contribute to the inflammatory cascade in the skin. These cytokines play a key role in the recruitment and activation of immune cells, leading to sustained inflammation and tissue damage.

Treatment Approaches: Modern medical treatments for psoriasis aim to alleviate symptoms, reduce inflammation, and slow down the abnormal skin cell turnover. Treatment options include topical medications (such as corticosteroids, vitamin D analogs, and retinoids), phototherapy (exposure to ultraviolet light), systemic medications (such as methotrexate, cyclosporine, and biologic agents targeting specific immune pathways), and oral retinoids.

Lifestyle Modifications: Lifestyle modifications such as stress management, maintaining a healthy weight, avoiding triggers, and adopting a balanced diet rich in fruits, vegetables, and omega-3 fatty acids may help in managing psoriasis symptoms and reducing flare-ups.

While modern medicine offers effective treatments for psoriasis, it is essential for individuals with psoriasis to work closely with healthcare professionals to develop a personalized treatment plan tailored to their specific needs and preferences. Additionally, ongoing research into the underlying mechanisms of psoriasis continues to improve our understanding of the condition and develop new therapeutic approaches.

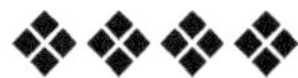

PITYRIASIS (सीप)

Pityriasis According to Ayurveda

Pityriasis, known as " सीप " in Ayurveda, is a skin condition characterized by the presence of patches of red, scaly skin.

In Ayurveda, the skin is considered a reflection of the overall health of an individual. When there is an imbalance in the doshas, it can manifest as skin disorders such as pityriasis

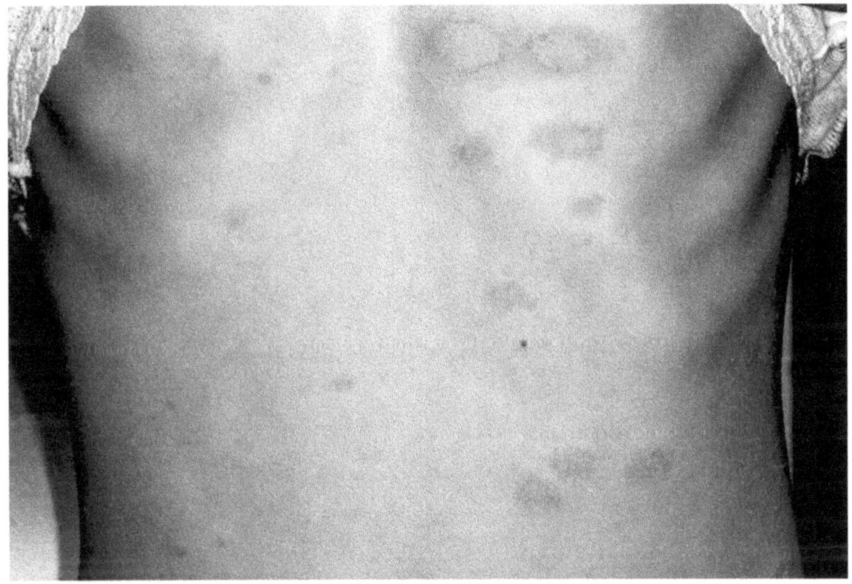

Dosha Imbalance: Ayurveda identifies specific doshic imbalances that contribute to the development of pityriasis. Imbalances in Pitta dosha are often associated with inflammation, heat, and redness, which can exacerbate skin conditions like pityriasis. Excess Vata dosha can lead to dryness and flakiness of the skin, while Kapha imbalance may result in excess oiliness and congestion.

Agni (Digestive Fire) Impairment: Ayurveda emphasizes the importance of balanced agni for overall health, including skin health. Impaired digestive fire can lead to the accumulation of ama, or toxins, in the body, which can manifest as skin disorders like pityriasis. Poor digestion and metabolism can exacerbate doshic imbalances and contribute to the development of skin conditions.

Diet and Lifestyle Factors: Ayurveda recognizes the influence of diet and lifestyle on skin health. Consuming foods that aggravate Pitta dosha, such as spicy, sour, and salty foods, can exacerbate inflammation and contribute to skin disorders. Similarly, unhealthy lifestyle habits like excessive stress, lack of sleep, and inadequate hydration can further imbalance the doshas and impact skin health.

Herbal Remedies: Ayurveda offers a variety of herbal remedies for managing pityriasis and restoring skin health. These may include herbs with cooling and soothing properties to pacify Pitta dosha, such as neem, aloe vera, and sandalwood. Additionally, herbs with purifying and detoxifying effects, such as turmeric, triphala, and manjistha, can help eliminate ama and promote clear, healthy skin.

Panchakarma Therapy: Panchakarma, a comprehensive detoxification therapy in Ayurveda, can be beneficial for addressing pityriasis and other skin disorders. Panchakarma treatments like Virechana (therapeutic purgation) and Raktamokshana (bloodletting) help eliminate accumulated toxins from the body, purify the blood, and balance the doshas. These therapies can be customized based on an individual's constitution and specific imbalances.

Balancing The Mind-Body Connection: Ayurveda recognizes the interconnectedness of the mind and body in health and disease. Stress, anxiety, and other emotional factors can influence skin health and exacerbate skin conditions like pityriasis. Practices such as yoga, meditation, and pranayama (breathwork) can help balance the mind-body connection, reduce stress, and support overall well-being, including skin health.

Pityriasis in Modern Medicine

In modern medicine, pityriasis refers to a group of skin conditions characterized by the formation of small, scaly patches on the skin. There are several types of pityriasis, each with its own distinct characteristics and causes. Here's an overview of pityriasis from a modern medical perspective:

Pityriasis Rosea: This is one of the most common forms of pityriasis. It typically begins with a single, large, pink or red patch, known as a "herald patch," followed by the appearance of smaller, scaly patches on the trunk, arms, and legs. The exact cause of pityriasis rosea is not known, but it is believed to be associated with viral infections, particularly the herpes virus.

Pityriasis Versicolor: Also known as "tinea versicolor," this form of pityriasis is caused by a yeast-like fungus called Malassezia. It is characterized by the presence of discolored patches on the skin, which may be lighter or darker than the surrounding skin. Pityriasis versicolor often occurs in areas of the body with high levels of sebum production, such as the chest, back, and shoulders.

Pityriasis Alba: This type of pityriasis is most commonly seen in children and adolescents. It is characterized by the presence of pale, scaly patches on the face, particularly on the cheeks. Pityriasis alba is thought to be a mild form of eczema, and its exact cause is not fully understood.

Pityriasis Rubra Pilaris: This is a rare and chronic skin disorder characterized by the presence of reddish-orange scaling patches and small, follicular papules. Pityriasis rubra pilaris can affect large areas of the body and may be associated with other medical conditions, such as autoimmune disorders.

Treatment: Treatment for pityriasis depends on the specific type and severity of the condition. In many cases, topical antifungal medications, such as ketoconazole or selenium sulfide, are used to treat pityriasis versicolor. For pityriasis rosea, treatment may involve the use of topical corticosteroids or oral antihistamines to alleviate itching and inflammation. Pityriasis alba often resolves on its own without treatment, but moisturizers and mild topical steroids may be recommended to alleviate symptoms. Pityriasis rubra pilaris may require more aggressive treatment, including systemic medications such as retinoids or immunosuppressants.

RAYNAUD'S PHENOMENON

Raynaud's Phenomenon According to Ayurveda

Raynaud's phenomenon is a condition characterized by episodic constriction of small arteries, typically in the fingers and toes, in response to cold or stress, leading to reduced blood flow and color changes in the affected areas. While Ayurveda doesn't have a specific term for Raynaud's phenomenon, it does provide insights into the underlying imbalances and potential remedies.

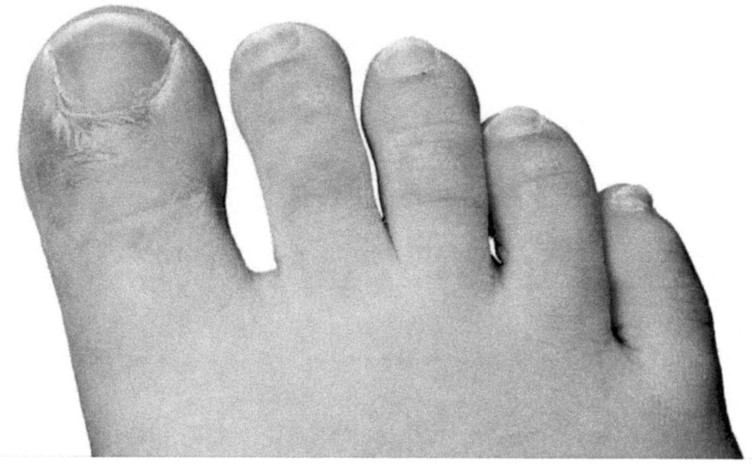

According to Ayurveda, Raynaud's phenomenon can be attributed to an imbalance in the Vata dosha, which governs movement and circulation in the body. When Vata is aggravated, it can lead to poor circulation and sensitivity to cold, both of which are characteristic features of Raynaud's.

To address Raynaud's phenomenon from an Ayurvedic perspective, the following principles and remedies can be considered:

Balancing Vata Dosha: Ayurveda emphasizes the importance of balancing the doshas to maintain overall health and well-being. This can be achieved through lifestyle modifications, including following a Vata-pacifying diet and daily routine. Warm, nourishing foods and drinks, such as soups, stews, herbal teas, and warm spices, can help pacify Vata and improve circulation.

Herbal Remedies: Ayurveda offers a range of herbs and herbal formulations that can support circulation and alleviate symptoms associated with Raynaud's phenomenon. Some herbs that are commonly used include ginger, turmeric, cinnamon, ashwagandha, and guggulu. These herbs have warming and circulatory-stimulating properties, which can help improve blood flow to the extremities.

Abhyanga (Ayurvedic Massage): Abhyanga, or self-massage with warm oil, is a therapeutic practice in Ayurveda that helps balance the doshas, improve circulation, and promote relaxation. Massaging the hands and feet with warm sesame oil or herbal oils can help alleviate symptoms of Raynaud's by enhancing blood flow to the affected areas.

Yoga and Pranayama: Gentle yoga poses and pranayama (breathing exercises) can help improve circulation, reduce stress, and balance the nervous system, all of which are beneficial for individuals with Raynaud's phenomenon. Poses that focus on opening the chest, stretching the hands and feet, and promoting relaxation can be particularly helpful.

Avoiding Cold and Stress: Since cold temperatures and stress can trigger episodes of Raynaud's phenomenon, it's important for individuals with this condition to avoid exposure to cold environments and manage stress effectively. Keeping the hands and feet warm, wearing gloves and socks, and practicing stress-reduction techniques such as meditation, mindfulness, and gentle exercise can all help prevent and manage symptoms.

Consultation with an Ayurvedic Practitioner: It's advisable for individuals with Raynaud's phenomenon to consult with a qualified Ayurvedic practitioner who can assess their unique constitution (prakriti) and imbalances, and recommend personalized treatment strategies based on their individual needs and health goals.

Raynaud's Phenomenon in Modern Medicine

Raynaud's phenomenon, a condition characterized by episodic constriction of small arteries in response to cold or stress, is primarily viewed and treated in modern medicine through the lens of vascular dysfunction and neurovascular regulation. Here's a detailed overview of Raynaud's phenomenon from a modern medical perspective:

Pathophysiology: Raynaud's phenomenon is believed to result from exaggerated vasoconstriction of the small arteries and arterioles in response to cold or emotional stress. This leads to a decrease in blood flow to the affected areas, typically the fingers and toes, causing pallor, followed by cyanosis (bluish discoloration), and finally, reactive hyperemia (redness) as blood flow is restored. The exact cause of this abnormal vascular response is not fully understood, but it is thought to involve dysregulation of the sympathetic nervous system and abnormalities in the endothelial cells lining the blood vessels.

Classification: Raynaud's phenomenon is classified into two main types: primary and secondary. Primary Raynaud's phenomenon, also known as Raynaud's disease, occurs in the absence of any underlying medical condition and is more common. Secondary Raynaud's phenomenon is associated with underlying conditions such as autoimmune diseases (e.g., systemic sclerosis), connective tissue disorders, vascular diseases, and certain medications.

Clinical Presentation: The hallmark of Raynaud's phenomenon is the triphasic color change of the affected digits: pallor, cyanosis, and reactive hyperemia. Patients may also experience pain, numbness, tingling, and cold sensation in the affected areas during episodes. The frequency and severity of episodes can vary widely among individuals, ranging from occasional mild episodes to frequent and severe attacks that significantly impact quality of life.

Diagnosis: Diagnosis of Raynaud's phenomenon is based on clinical presentation and history, including a detailed assessment of symptoms, triggers, and associated medical conditions. In some cases, additional tests may be performed to rule out underlying secondary causes, such as blood tests for autoimmune markers, nailfold capillaroscopy to assess microvascular abnormalities, and imaging studies to evaluate blood flow.

Treatment: The management of Raynaud's phenomenon aims to alleviate symptoms, prevent complications, and improve quality of life. Treatment strategies may include lifestyle modifications (e.g., avoiding cold exposure, wearing warm clothing), pharmacotherapy (e.g., calcium channel blockers, vasodilators), and biofeedback techniques to control sympathetic nervous system activity. In cases of secondary Raynaud's phenomenon, treatment is directed toward addressing the underlying cause.

Prognosis: The prognosis of Raynaud's phenomenon depends on its underlying cause and severity. In most cases, primary Raynaud's phenomenon has a benign course with relatively mild symptoms that can be managed effectively with conservative measures. However, secondary Raynaud's phenomenon, especially when associated with systemic diseases, may have a more variable prognosis and require more aggressive treatment and monitoring.

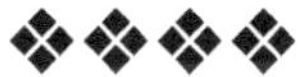

RINGWORM

Ringworm According to Ayurveda

Ringworm, known in Ayurveda as "dadru," is a common fungal infection of the skin Ayurvedic texts describe ringworm as a condition that affects the skin, leading to symptoms such as itching, redness, and the appearance of circular lesions.

According to Ayurveda, the primary cause of ringworm is the vitiation of the pitta and kapha doshas. Pitta represents the fire element and is responsible for metabolism and digestion, while kapha represents the earth and water elements and governs structure and lubrication in the body. When there is an imbalance in these doshas, it can lead to the accumulation of toxins in the body, which in turn can manifest as skin disorders such as ringworm.

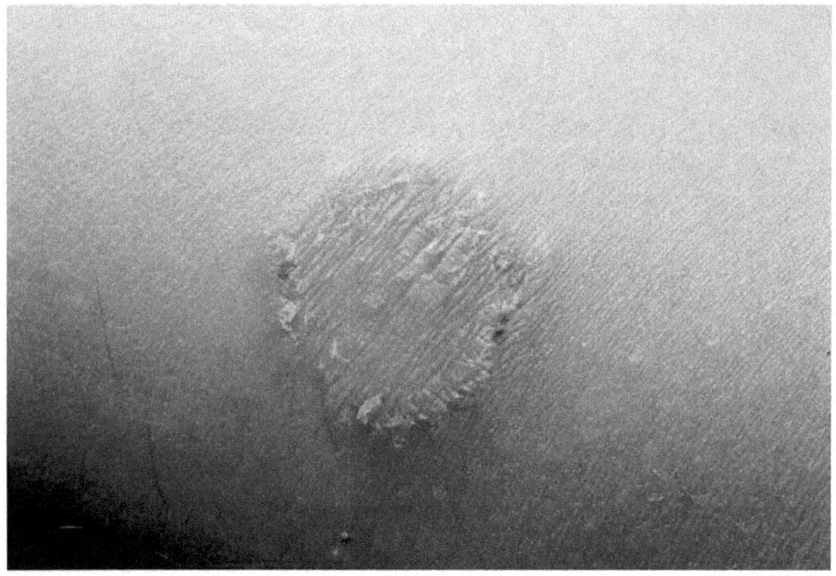

Ayurvedic treatment for ringworm focuses on restoring the balance of the doshas and eliminating toxins from the body.

Dietary recommendations for individuals with ringworm include avoiding spicy, oily, and fried foods, as these can aggravate the pitta dosha and worsen symptoms. Instead, a diet rich in cooling and nourishing foods, such as fresh fruits and vegetables, whole grains, and herbal teas, is recommended to pacify the aggravated doshas and support healing.

Lifestyle modifications play a crucial role in the management of ringworm according to Ayurveda. Practices such as maintaining proper hygiene, keeping the affected area clean and dry, and avoiding sharing personal items such as towels and clothing can help prevent the spread of the infection and promote healing.

Herbal remedies are an integral part of Ayurvedic treatment for ringworm. Commonly used herbs include neem (Azadirachta indica), turmeric (Curcuma longa), aloe vera (Aloe barbadensis), and tulsi (Ocimum sanctum). These herbs possess anti-fungal, anti-inflammatory, and cooling properties, which help to soothe the skin, reduce inflammation, and eliminate the fungus responsible for ringworm.

Ayurvedic treatment for ringworm may also include external therapies such as herbal pastes, medicated oils, and herbal baths. These therapies are designed to cleanse and nourish the skin, promote healing, and prevent recurrence of the infection.

Ringworm in Modern Medicine

In modern medicine, ringworm is known as dermatophytosis, and it is a fungal infection of the skin caused by various species of fungi called dermatophytes. Unlike Ayurveda, which attributes ringworm to doshic imbalances, modern medicine identifies specific fungal pathogens as the primary cause of the infection.

Dermatophytes thrive in warm, moist environments and can infect the skin, nails, and hair. Ringworm typically presents as circular or ring-shaped lesions on the skin, which may be red, scaly, and itchy. The infection can spread through direct contact with an infected person or animal, as well as through contact with contaminated surfaces such as towels, clothing, and sports equipment.

Diagnosis of ringworm in modern medicine often involves clinical evaluation of the skin lesions and may include microscopic examination of skin scrapings or fungal cultures to identify the specific type of fungus causing the infection.

Treatment of ringworm in modern medicine typically involves the use of antifungal medications, which may be applied topically as creams, ointments, or sprays, or taken orally as tablets or capsules. Common antifungal agents used to treat ringworm include clotrimazole, miconazole, terbinafine, and fluconazole. These medications work by inhibiting the growth and reproduction of the fungus, thereby resolving the infection.

In addition to antifungal medications, maintaining proper hygiene and keeping the affected area clean and dry are essential aspects of managing ringworm in modern medicine. It is also important to avoid sharing personal items such as towels, clothing, and grooming tools to prevent the spread of the infection.

In cases of severe or recurrent ringworm infections, a healthcare provider may recommend additional treatments such as phototherapy (light therapy) or systemic antifungal medications.

Overall, modern medicine offers effective treatments for ringworm, focusing on the use of antifungal medications to eliminate the fungal infection and promote healing of the skin. With proper diagnosis and treatment, most cases of ringworm can be successfully managed, and recurrence can be prevented with good hygiene practices.

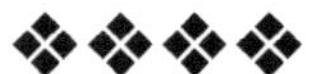

ROSACEA (रोजेशिया)

Rosacea According to Ayurveda

Rosacea, known as "रोजेशिया" in Ayurveda, is a chronic skin condition that primarily affects the face, characterized by redness, visible blood vessels, and sometimes pimples and swelling. In Ayurveda, rosacea is understood as a Pitta dosha imbalance primarily, with involvement of other doshas as well.

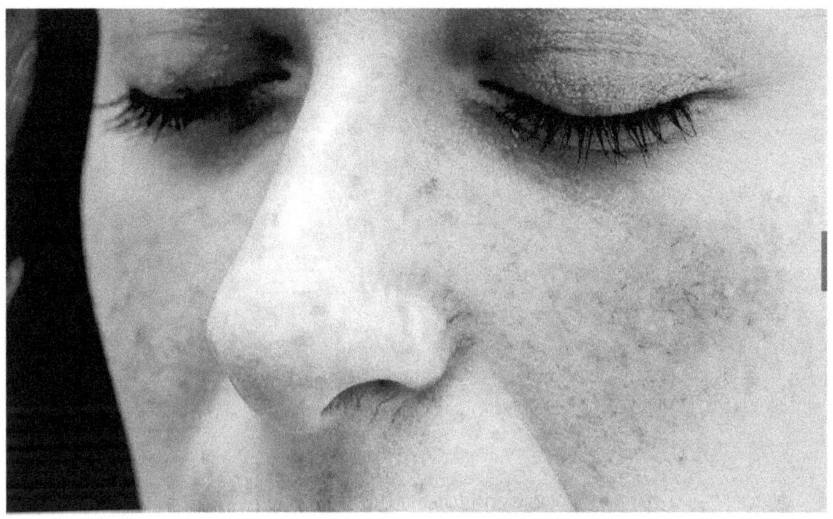

Pitta Imbalance: Pitta dosha governs heat, metabolism, and digestion. Excessive consumption of Pitta-aggravating foods such as spicy, oily, fried, and acidic foods can lead to an imbalance in Pitta dosha, which manifests as inflammation and heat in the skin, contributing to rosacea symptoms.

Ama Formation: In Ayurveda, ama refers to toxins formed as a result of poor digestion and metabolism. When the digestive fire (agni) is weak, undigested food particles (ama) accumulate in the body, leading to various health issues, including skin disorders like rosacea.

Sensitivity to Triggers: Individuals with rosacea often have triggers that exacerbate their symptoms, such as sun exposure, stress, alcohol, hot beverages, and certain skincare products. Ayurveda emphasizes understanding individual constitution (prakriti) and identifying triggers that disturb the dosha balance.

Emotional Factors: Emotional stress and disturbances can aggravate Pitta dosha and contribute to rosacea flare-ups. Ayurveda recommends practices like meditation, yoga, and pranayama to calm the mind and reduce stress.

Impaired Liver Function: According to Ayurveda, the liver (yakrit) plays a crucial role in detoxification and maintaining healthy skin. Impaired liver function can lead to the accumulation of toxins in the body, worsening rosacea symptoms.

Treatment of rosacea in Ayurveda focuses on addressing the root cause of the condition and restoring dosha balance. Here are some Ayurvedic recommendations for managing rosacea:

Dietary Modifications: Follow a Pitta-pacifying diet by consuming cooling and soothing foods such as fresh fruits, vegetables, whole grains, dairy products, and herbal teas. Avoid Pitta-aggravating foods like spicy, sour, and fried items.

Herbal Remedies: Ayurvedic herbs such as neem, turmeric, manjistha, and aloe vera have cooling and anti-inflammatory properties that can help alleviate rosacea symptoms when used topically or internally.

Detoxification: Panchakarma, a detoxification therapy in Ayurveda, can help eliminate ama and toxins from the body, thereby reducing inflammation and improving skin health.

Stress Management: Practice stress-reducing techniques such as meditation, yoga, and deep breathing exercises to keep Pitta dosha in balance and prevent stress-related flare-ups.

Skincare Routine: Use gentle and natural skincare products suitable for sensitive skin. Avoid harsh chemicals, fragrances, and abrasive exfoliants that can irritate the skin and worsen rosacea symptoms.

Lifestyle Modifications: Maintain a regular daily routine, get an adequate amount of sleep, and avoid excessive sun exposure and heat.

Rosacea in Modern Medicine

Rosacea, known as "रोजेशिया" in Hindi, is a common chronic skin condition that primarily affects the face. In modern medicine, rosacea is understood as a multifactorial disorder involving a combination of genetic, environmental, vascular, inflammatory, and microbial factors. While the exact cause of rosacea remains unclear, several contributing factors and potential triggers have been identified:

Genetics: There is evidence to suggest that rosacea may have a genetic component, as it tends to run in families.

Dysregulation of The Immune System: Dysfunctions in the immune system may contribute to the inflammation seen in rosacea, although the precise mechanisms are still being studied.

Demodex Mites: These microscopic mites that inhabit the skin may play a role in the development of rosacea, particularly in individuals with an overabundance of these mites.

Vascular Abnormalities: Blood vessel abnormalities, including dilation and increased permeability, are characteristic features of rosacea. These abnormalities contribute to the persistent redness and flushing seen in affected individuals.

Environmental Triggers: Various environmental factors can exacerbate rosacea symptoms, including sun exposure, temperature extremes, wind, humidity, certain skincare products, spicy foods, alcohol, and stress.

Microbial Factors: While not fully understood, certain microorganisms, including bacteria and mites, may play a role in the pathogenesis of rosacea.

The clinical presentation of rosacea can vary widely among individuals and may include:

Persistent facial redness, particularly in the central part of the face
Flushing or transient redness triggered by various factors
Visible blood vessels (telangiectasia)
Papules and pustules resembling acne, particularly in subtype 2 (papulopustular rosacea)
Thickening of the skin, particularly in advanced cases (phymatous rosacea)
Treatment options for rosacea in modern medicine aim to control symptoms, reduce inflammation, and improve the overall appearance of the skin. These may include:

Topical Therapies: Topical medications such as metronidazole, azelaic acid, and brimonidine may help reduce redness, inflammation, and the appearance of papules and pustules.

Oral Medications: Oral antibiotics (e.g., doxycycline, minocycline) may be prescribed to reduce inflammation and control bacterial overgrowth on the skin.

Laser and Light Therapies: Various laser and light-based treatments can target blood vessels, reduce redness, and improve the appearance of telangiectasia and erythema.

Skincare and Sun Protection: Gentle skincare products and sun protection are essential for managing rosacea and minimizing flare-ups.

Avoiding Triggers: Identifying and avoiding triggers that exacerbate rosacea symptoms can help minimize flare-ups and improve symptom control.

In severe cases, surgical interventions such as dermabrasion or laser therapy may be considered to address thickened skin and other disfigurements associated with phymatous rosacea.

It's important for individuals with rosacea to work closely with a dermatologist to develop a personalized treatment plan tailored to their specific needs and symptoms. Regular follow-up appointments and adjustments to treatment may be necessary to achieve optimal control of the condition.

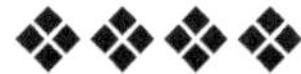

Scabies According to Ayurveda

Scabies, known as "Pama" in Ayurveda, is a skin condition caused by the infestation of the Sarcoptes scabiei mite. According to Ayurveda, Pama is primarily caused by an imbalance of the Vata and Kapha doshas, leading to symptoms like intense itching, redness, and the appearance of small, raised bumps or blisters on the skin. Let's delve deeper into Ayurvedic understanding and treatment of Pama:

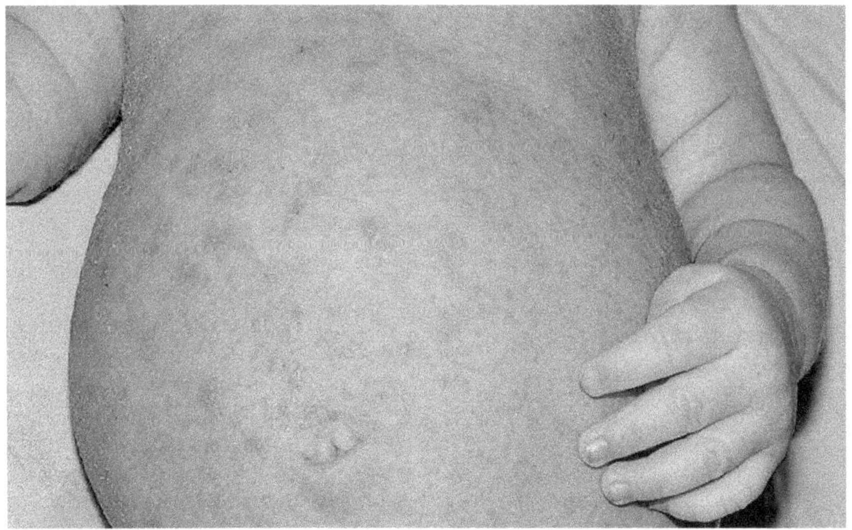

Understanding Pama (Scabies) In Ayurveda:

Dosha Imbalance: Ayurveda views Pama as primarily arising from an aggravation of Vata and Kapha doshas. Vata imbalance leads to dryness, roughness, and itching, while Kapha imbalance causes the formation of mucus and fluid-filled lesions on the skin.

Ama Formation: The accumulation of toxins (ama) in the body due to improper digestion and metabolism can also contribute to the development of Pama. Ama blocks the channels of circulation and nourishment, leading to skin inflammation and itching.

Contagious Nature: Ayurveda recognizes Pama as a contagious condition, often spread through direct skin contact with an infected individual or through sharing contaminated objects like clothing, towels, or bedding.

Symptoms of Pama (Scabies) In Ayurveda:

Severe Itching: One of the hallmark symptoms of Pama is intense itching, especially at night or after a hot shower, which worsens with scratching.

Skin Lesions: Infestation by the Sarcoptes scabiei mite leads to the formation of small, raised bumps, vesicles, or pustules on the skin. These lesions may appear in clusters, particularly in areas with thin skin such as between the fingers, wrists, elbows, knees, and genitalia.

Redness and Inflammation: The affected skin may become red, inflamed, and tender due to scratching and the body's immune response to the mite infestation.

Secondary Infections: Continuous scratching can break the skin barrier, increasing the risk of secondary bacterial infections and complications.

Ayurvedic Management of Pama (Scabies):

Balancing Doshas: Treatment aims at pacifying the aggravated Vata and Kapha doshas through dietary and lifestyle modifications. This includes consuming warm, nourishing foods and herbs that are anti-inflammatory and soothing to the skin.

Detoxification: Ayurvedic therapies such as Panchakarma (cleansing procedures) help eliminate ama from the body and restore proper digestion and metabolism.

Topical Remedies: Herbal pastes, oils, or powders containing ingredients like neem, turmeric, and Sariva (Hemidesmus indicus) are applied topically to relieve itching, reduce inflammation, and kill the mites.

Internal Medications: Ayurvedic practitioners may prescribe internal medicines like Triphala, Gandhak Rasayana, and Sarivadyasava to purify the blood, boost immunity, and eliminate parasites from the body.

Hygiene Practices: Maintaining personal hygiene, avoiding sharing personal items, and regularly washing clothes and bedding in hot water are essential to prevent the spread of Pama.

Scabies in Modern Medicine

In modern medicine, scabies is recognized as a contagious skin infestation caused by the Sarcoptes scabiei mite. Here's an overview of scabies from the perspective of modern medicine:

Etiology and Pathogenesis: Scabies is caused by the burrowing of the female Sarcoptes scabiei mite into the superficial layers of the skin, where it lays eggs. The infestation typically occurs through prolonged skin-to-skin contact with an infected person. The mite's saliva, feces, and eggs trigger an allergic reaction in the skin, leading to intense itching and inflammation.

Clinical Presentation: The primary symptom of scabies is severe itching, which often worsens at night or after a hot shower. Other common symptoms include:

Skin Lesions: Small, raised bumps, vesicles, or pustules may appear on the skin, especially in areas such as the wrists, elbows, armpits, genitalia, and webbing between the fingers.

Redness and Inflammation: The affected skin may become red, swollen, and tender due to scratching and the body's immune response to the mite infestation.

Secondary Infections: Continuous scratching can lead to breaks in the skin, increasing the risk of bacterial infections and complications.

Diagnosis: Scabies is typically diagnosed based on clinical presentation and history of exposure to an infected individual. In some cases, a skin scraping or biopsy may be performed to identify the mites, eggs, or fecal matter under a microscope.

Treatment: The standard treatment for scabies in modern medicine involves topical medications and, in some cases, oral medications. Common treatment options include:

Topical Scabicides: Permethrin cream or lotion is the most commonly prescribed topical treatment for scabies. It is applied to the entire body from the neck down and left on for a specified period before washing off. Other options include sulfur ointment, crotamiton cream, or benzyl benzoate lotion.

Oral Medications: In severe cases or when topical treatments fail, oral medications such as ivermectin may be prescribed. Ivermectin is an antiparasitic medication that helps kill the scabies mites.

Treatment of Complications: Secondary bacterial infections may require antibiotic treatment to resolve.

Prevention: Preventing the spread of scabies involves:

Avoiding Close Contact: Minimize skin-to-skin contact with infected individuals.

Personal Hygiene: Maintain good personal hygiene, including regular handwashing and bathing.

Environmental Measures: Wash Clothes, Bedding, And Towels in Hot Water to kill any mites or eggs.

STOMATITIS (मुखपाक)

Stomatitis According to Ayurveda

Stomatitis, according to Ayurveda, is known as "Mukhapaka." In Ayurvedic terms, it refers to inflammation of the oral mucosa, often accompanied by pain, redness, swelling, and sometimes ulceration.

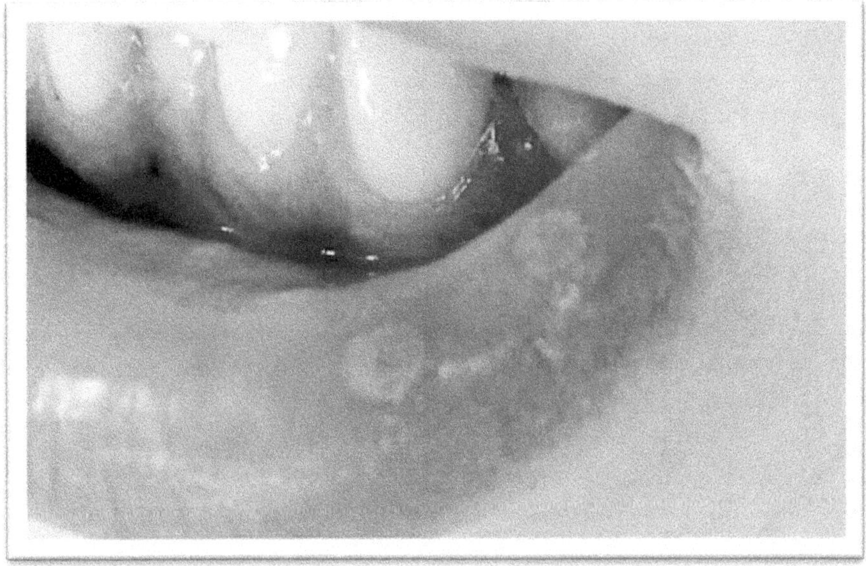

Stomatitis Can Be Classified into Different Types Based On the Dosha Involvement:

Vata-Type Stomatitis: This type is characterized by symptoms such as dryness, cracking, and pain in the oral cavity. Vata imbalance leads to decreased saliva production, which can cause dryness and discomfort. To treat Vata-type stomatitis, Ayurveda suggests the use of lubricating oils or ghee (clarified butter) for oral application, along with internal consumption of nourishing, oily foods to balance Vata dosha.

Pitta-Type Stomatitis: Pitta dominance manifests as inflammation, redness, and burning sensation in the mouth. Pitta aggravation can be caused by excessive intake of spicy, hot, and acidic foods, as well as emotional stress.

Ayurvedic treatment for Pitta-type stomatitis involves cooling and soothing remedies such as herbal mouth rinses made from herbs like licorice (Yashtimadhu) and coriander (Dhanyaka). Pitta-pacifying diet and lifestyle modifications are also recommended to alleviate symptoms.

Kapha-Type Stomatitis: Kapha imbalance results in excessive salivation, thick mucus formation, and a feeling of heaviness in the mouth. This type of stomatitis is often associated with poor oral hygiene and the accumulation of toxins. Ayurvedic management of Kapha-type stomatitis includes herbal mouthwashes containing astringent and antimicrobial herbs like neem (Azadirachta indica) and Triphala churna (a combination of three fruits: Amalaki, Bibhitaki, and Haritaki). Kapha-balancing diet and practices to improve digestion are also recommended.

In addition to addressing the specific doshic imbalances, Ayurveda emphasizes the importance of detoxification and strengthening of the digestive system to prevent stomatitis recurrence. Panchakarma therapies such as Vamana (therapeutic emesis) and Virechana (therapeutic purgation) are recommended to eliminate accumulated toxins from the body. Following a Sattvic diet (balanced, wholesome, and easily digestible) and practicing oral hygiene rituals like oil pulling (Gandusha) with medicated oils are also beneficial in managing stomatitis.

Furthermore, Ayurveda considers the role of mental and emotional factors in the manifestation of stomatitis. Stress, anxiety, and emotional disturbances can aggravate doshic imbalances and weaken the immune system, making the individual more susceptible to oral health issues. Therefore, stress management techniques such as meditation, yoga, and pranayama (breathing exercises) are advocated to promote overall well-being and oral health.

Stomatitis in Modern Medicine

Stomatitis in modern medicine refers to inflammation of the mucous membrane lining the mouth, commonly characterized by symptoms such as pain, redness, swelling, and sometimes ulceration. There are several types of stomatitis, including:

Herpetic Stomatitis: Caused by the herpes simplex virus (HSV), this type of stomatitis presents with painful, fluid-filled blisters on the lips, inside the mouth, or around the gums. It is highly contagious and can recur periodically.

Aphthous Stomatitis (Canker Sores): Aphthous ulcers are small, painful lesions that can develop on the soft tissues inside the mouth, such as the tongue, inner cheeks, and lips. The exact cause is unknown, but factors such as stress, injury, hormonal changes, and certain foods may trigger their formation.

Chemotherapy-Induced Stomatitis: Some cancer treatments, particularly chemotherapy and radiation therapy, can damage the mucous membranes of the mouth, leading to stomatitis. Symptoms include pain, ulcers, and difficulty eating and swallowing.

Allergic Stomatitis: Allergic reactions to certain foods, medications, or dental materials can cause stomatitis symptoms, including swelling, redness, and ulceration in the mouth.

Bacterial or Fungal Stomatitis: Infections caused by bacteria or fungi, such as candidiasis (oral thrush) or bacterial infections like streptococcal stomatitis, can result in stomatitis symptoms.

Treatment for stomatitis in modern medicine depends on the underlying cause and severity of symptoms. It may include:

Topical Treatments: Antimicrobial mouthwashes, topical corticosteroids, or numbing agents (e.g., lidocaine) can help reduce pain and inflammation.

Systemic Medications: In cases of severe or recurrent stomatitis, oral medications such as antivirals (e.g., acyclovir for herpetic stomatitis), corticosteroids, or immunosuppressant may be prescribed.

Pain Management: Over-the-counter pain relievers (e.g., acetaminophen, ibuprofen) can help alleviate discomfort associated with stomatitis.

Preventive Measures: Practicing good oral hygiene, avoiding known triggers (such as certain foods or irritating substances), and maintaining a healthy lifestyle can help prevent stomatitis episodes.

n some cases, medical intervention may be necessary to address complications or underlying conditions contributing to stomatitis.

TINEA (फफूंदी)

Tinea According to Ayurveda

Tinea, commonly known as "Fafundi" in Ayurveda, is a fungal infection of the skin. According to Ayurveda, Tinea is primarily caused by an imbalance in the doshas, particularly the Pitta and Kapha doshas. When these doshas are aggravated, they weaken the skin's natural defenses, making it more susceptible to fungal infections.

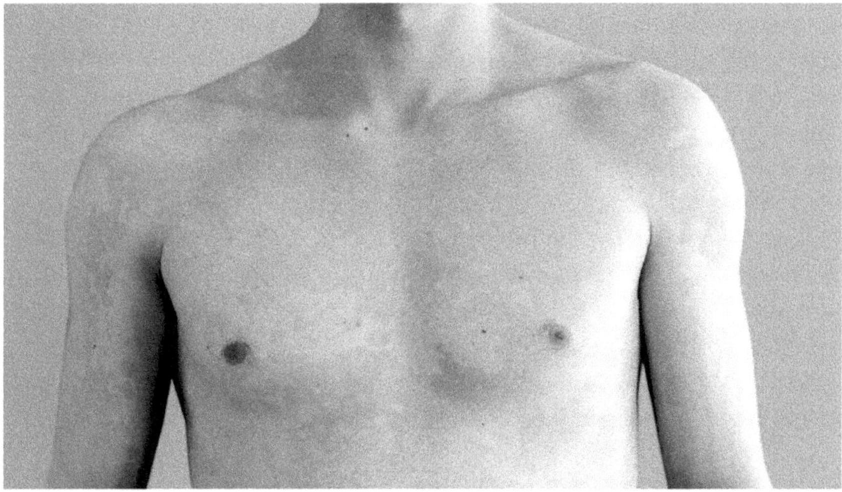

In Ayurveda, Tinea is categorized under "Kshudra Kushtha" (minor skin diseases) and is believed to be caused by factors such as excessive sweating, poor hygiene, consumption of excessive spicy and oily foods, and suppression of natural urges. These factors lead to the accumulation of toxins (ama) in the body, further exacerbating the condition.

Symptoms of Tinea according to Ayurveda include redness, itching, and circular patches on the skin, which may be accompanied by a burning sensation. Ayurvedic texts also describe different types of Tinea based on the predominant dosha involved:

Vata-Type Tinea: Characterized by dryness, roughness, and cracking of the skin. It may be associated with symptoms such as pain and itching.

Pitta-Type Tinea: Manifests as redness, inflammation, and a burning sensation on the affected area. The lesions may be warm to the touch and may ooze pus in severe cases.

Kapha-Type Tinea: Presents with thick, moist, and discolored patches on the skin. It may be accompanied by itching and a foul smell.

Ayurvedic treatment of Tinea aims to balance the aggravated doshas, eliminate toxins from the body, and strengthen the skin's natural defenses. The treatment approach typically includes:

Dietary and Lifestyle Modifications: Avoiding spicy, oily, and junk foods, maintaining proper hygiene, and following a balanced diet rich in fresh fruits, vegetables, and whole grains.

Internal Medications: Ayurvedic formulations containing herbs like Neem (Azadirachta indica), Haridra (Turmeric), Guduchi (Tinospora cordifolia), and Triphala (a combination of three fruits) are prescribed to purify the blood, boost immunity, and eliminate toxins from the body.

External Applications: Local applications of herbal pastes, oils, or powders containing ingredients like Neem, Turmeric, and Manjistha (Rubia cordifolia) help relieve itching, inflammation, and promote healing of the affected skin.

Panchakarma Therapy: In severe cases, Panchakarma procedures such as Virechana (therapeutic purgation) or Raktamokshana (bloodletting) may be recommended to eliminate toxins from the body and restore doshic balance.

Yoga and Pranayama: Regular practice of yoga asanas and pranayama (breathing exercises) helps reduce stress, improve blood circulation, and strengthen the immune system, which is beneficial in managing Tinea.

Tinea in Modern Medicine

In modern medicine, Tinea, also known as ringworm, is a fungal infection of the skin, hair, or nails caused by various species of dermatophyte fungi. It can affect people of all ages and is highly contagious. The common types of Tinea infections include Tinea corporis (ringworm of the body), Tinea cruris (jock itch), Tinea pedis (athlete's foot), and Tinea capitis (scalp ringworm).

The main causative agents of Tinea infections are fungi belonging to the genera Trichophyton, Microsporum, and Epidermophyton. These fungi thrive in warm, moist environments and can spread through direct contact with an infected person or contaminated objects such as towels, clothing, and surfaces.

Symptoms of Tinea infections typically include red, scaly patches on the skin, which may be itchy and have a raised border. In Tinea capitis, hair loss and scalp inflammation may also occur. Diagnosis is usually made based on clinical presentation and confirmed through laboratory tests such as microscopic examination of skin scrapings or fungal cultures.

Treatment of Tinea infections in modern medicine involves antifungal medications, which may be applied topically as creams, lotions, or powders for mild cases, or taken orally for more severe or widespread infections. Common antifungal agents used include clotrimazole, miconazole, terbinafine, and fluconazole. Additionally, keeping the affected area clean and dry, avoiding sharing personal items, and wearing loose-fitting clothing can help prevent the spread and recurrence of Tinea infections.

It's important to note that while modern medicine focuses on treating the symptoms and eradicating the fungal infection, Ayurvedic medicine approaches Tinea from a holistic perspective, addressing underlying imbalances in the body's constitution and promoting overall health and well-being. Both approaches can complement each other in managing Tinea infections effectively.

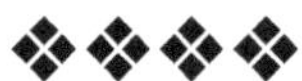

Urticaria According to Ayurveda

In Ayurveda, Urticaria, known as "Sheetapitta," is a condition characterized by sudden onset of raised, itchy, and reddish welts or hives on the skin. According to Ayurvedic principles, Sheetapitta is primarily caused by an imbalance in the Pitta dosha, aggravated by factors such as improper diet, stress, environmental toxins, and incompatible food combinations.

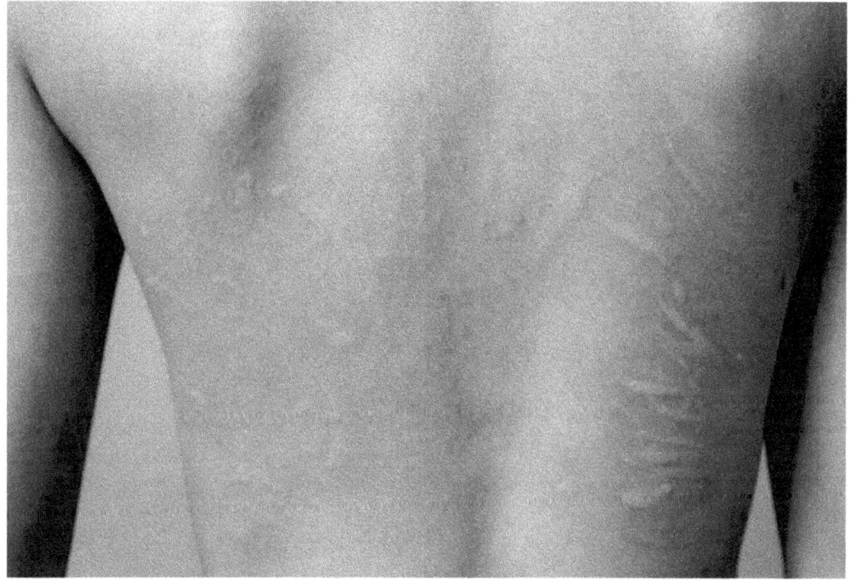

According to Ayurveda, Sheetapitta occurs due to an imbalance in the Pitta dosha, which governs metabolism, digestion, and transformation in the body. Pitta aggravation can lead to excessive heat in the body, causing inflammation and skin reactions. The vitiated Pitta combines with the impurities in the body (ama) and circulates in the blood, manifesting as Sheetapitta on the skin.

Etiology: Several factors can contribute to the aggravation of Pitta dosha and the onset of Sheetapitta:

Improper Diet: Consuming excessively spicy, oily, acidic, or sour foods can aggravate Pitta dosha and contribute to the development of Sheetapitta.

Emotional Stress: Emotional factors such as anxiety, anger, and stress can disturb the balance of doshas in the body, particularly Pitta, leading to skin disorders like Urticaria.

Environmental Toxins: Exposure to environmental pollutants, chemicals, and allergens can trigger allergic reactions in susceptible individuals, manifesting as hives or welts.

Incompatible Food Combinations: Consuming incompatible food combinations, such as milk with fish or fruit with dairy, can create toxins in the body and aggravate Pitta dosha, contributing to Sheetapitta.

Symptoms: The main symptoms of Sheetapitta include:

Reddish, raised welts or hives on the skin
Intense itching and burning sensation
Swelling and inflammation of the affected area
Sensitivity to heat and sunlight
Aggravation of symptoms after consuming spicy or acidic foods

Ayurvedic Management: Ayurvedic treatment for Sheetapitta focuses on pacifying the aggravated Pitta dosha, eliminating toxins from the body, and restoring the balance of doshas. The treatment approach includes:

Diet and Lifestyle Modifications:

Avoiding spicy, sour, and acidic foods

Consuming cooling and Pitta-pacifying foods such as sweet fruits, vegetables, and grains

Practicing stress-reducing techniques such as yoga, meditation, and pranayama

Protecting the skin from excessive heat and sunlight exposure

Herbal Remedies: Ayurvedic herbs such as Neem (Azadirachta indica), Aloe vera, Turmeric (Curcuma longa), and Manjistha (Rubia cordifolia) are beneficial in reducing inflammation, itching, and purifying the blood.

Detoxification Therapies: Panchakarma therapies such as Virechana (therapeutic purgation) and Raktamokshana (bloodletting) are effective in eliminating toxins from the body and balancing Pitta dosha.

External Applications: Application of cooling and soothing herbal pastes or oils on the affected skin can provide relief from itching and inflammation.

Urticaria in Modern Medicine

Urticaria, known as "शीतपित्त" in Ayurveda, is termed similarly in Modern Medicine. Urticaria is a skin condition characterized by the sudden appearance of raised, itchy, and reddish welts or hives. In Modern Medicine, Urticaria is primarily classified into two types: acute and chronic.

Acute Urticarla: Acute Urticaria typically lasts for less than six weeks and is often caused by allergic reactions to foods, medications, insect stings, or environmental factors such as pollen or pet dander.

Other triggers may include infections, stress, and exposure to heat or cold.

Acute Urticaria usually resolves on its own or with antihistamine medications to relieve itching and inflammation.

Chronic Urticaria: Chronic Urticaria lasts for more than six weeks and may persist for months or even years.

The exact cause of chronic Urticaria is often more challenging to identify and may involve autoimmune factors, underlying medical conditions, or idiopathic mechanisms.

Treatment for chronic Urticaria typically involves a combination of antihistamines, corticosteroids, and other medications to manage symptoms and reduce inflammation.

TREATMENT APPROACHES:

Antihistamines: These medications block the action of histamine, a chemical released during allergic reactions, to reduce itching and inflammation.

Corticosteroids: In severe cases, corticosteroids may be prescribed to suppress the immune response and reduce inflammation.

Avoiding Triggers: Identifying and avoiding triggers such as specific foods, medications, or environmental allergens can help prevent Urticaria outbreaks.

Other Therapies: In cases of chronic Urticaria, additional treatments such as omalizumab (an anti-IgE antibody) or immunosuppressive agents may be considered to manage symptoms.

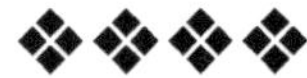

VITILIGO (श्वेतकुष्ठ)

Vitiligo According to Ayurveda

Vitiligo, known as "श्वेतकुष्ठ" (Shwetakushtha) in Ayurveda, is a condition characterized by the loss of skin pigmentation, resulting in white patches on the skin. It is classified under the category of Kushtha (skin diseases) in Ayurveda.

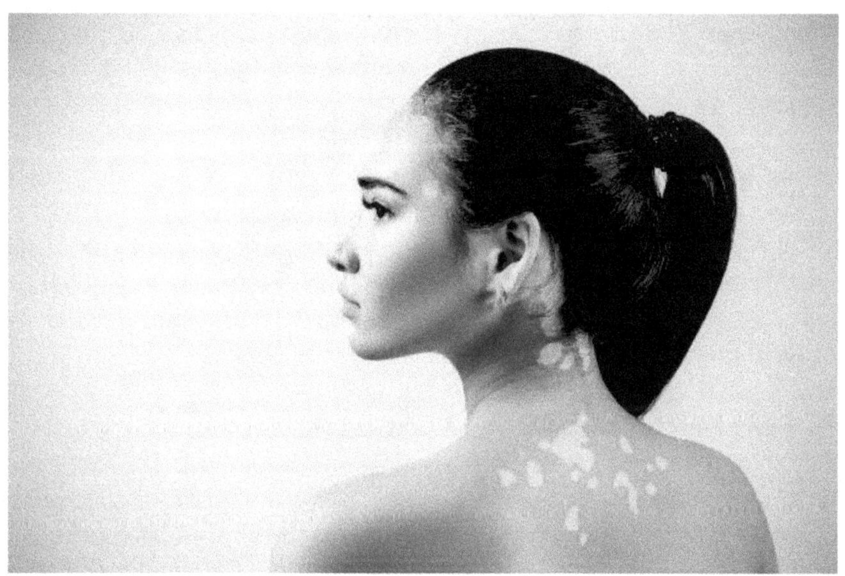

In Ayurvedic philosophy, the body is believed to be composed of three doshas: Vata, Pitta, and Kapha. Vitiligo is primarily associated with an aggravated Pitta dosha, which leads to the destruction of melanocytes (pigment-producing cells) in the skin. Kapha imbalance can also contribute to the manifestation of vitiligo by obstructing the channels of nutrition to the skin.

Ayurveda emphasizes the importance of treating vitiligo holistically, addressing both the underlying imbalance in the doshas and the manifestation of symptoms on the skin.

Pitta Pacifying Therapies: Ayurvedic treatments for vitiligo focus on pacifying the aggravated Pitta dosha. This may involve the use of cooling herbs and formulations such as Aloe vera, Neem (Azadirachta indica), Manjistha (Rubia cordifolia), and Guduchi (Tinospora cordifolia). These herbs help to detoxify the body and cool down the excessive heat associated with Pitta imbalance.

Blood Purification: Since vitiligo is considered a disorder of the blood and skin tissues, Ayurvedic therapies often aim to purify the blood and remove toxins from the body. This can be achieved through the use of blood-purifying herbs such as Sariva (Hemidesmus indicus), Triphala (a combination of three fruits: Amalaki, Bibhitaki, and Haritaki), and Guggulu (Commiphora mukul).

External Therapies: Localized treatment of vitiligo patches is also important in Ayurveda. External therapies may include the application of herbal pastes, oils, and ointments to the affected areas. Some commonly used formulations include Mahatiktaka Ghrita, Bakuchi (Psoralea corylifolia) oil, and Chandanadi taila. These therapies help to stimulate melanocyte function and promote pigmentation in the affected areas.

Dietary and Lifestyle Modifications: Ayurveda emphasizes the importance of dietary and lifestyle factors in managing vitiligo. Patients are advised to avoid Pitta-aggravating foods such as spicy, sour, and acidic foods, as well as alcohol and tobacco. Instead, they are encouraged to consume cooling and nourishing foods such as fresh fruits, vegetables, whole grains, and dairy products. Stress management techniques, regular exercise, and adequate sleep are also important aspects of vitiligo management according to Ayurveda.

Panchakarma Therapy: In severe cases of vitiligo or when other treatment modalities fail, Ayurvedic practitioners may recommend Panchakarma therapy. Panchakarma is a comprehensive detoxification and rejuvenation therapy that involves various cleansing procedures to eliminate toxins from the body and restore balance to the doshas.

Vitiligo In Modern Medicine

In modern medicine, vitiligo is considered an autoimmune condition where the body's immune system mistakenly attacks and destroys melanocytes, the cells responsible for producing skin pigment. The exact cause of this autoimmune response is not fully understood, but it is believed to involve a combination of genetic, environmental, and immunological factors.

Autoimmune Response: The prevailing theory in modern medicine is that vitiligo occurs due to an autoimmune response, where the body's immune system mistakenly targets and destroys melanocytes. This leads to the loss of pigment in the affected areas of the skin.

Genetic Factors: There is evidence to suggest that genetic factors play a role in predisposing individuals to vitiligo. It often runs in families, and certain gene variations have been associated with an increased risk of developing the condition.

Environmental Triggers: While the exact environmental triggers are not fully understood, factors such as stress, exposure to certain chemicals, trauma to the skin, and sunburn have been implicated in triggering or exacerbating vitiligo in susceptible individuals.

Melanocyte Dysfunction: In addition to autoimmune destruction, abnormalities in melanocyte function have also been observed in vitiligo. This includes impaired melanocyte migration, proliferation, and survival in the affected areas of the skin.

Treatment Options: Modern medicine offers several treatment options for vitiligo, including topical corticosteroids, calcineurin inhibitors, phototherapy (such as narrowband UVB therapy), and surgical procedures like skin grafting and melanocyte transplantation. These treatments aim to repigment the affected areas of the skin and minimize the spread of vitiligo.

Psychosocial Impact: Vitiligo can have a significant psychosocial impact on affected individuals, leading to feelings of embarrassment, low self-esteem, and social isolation. Counseling and support groups may be beneficial in helping individuals cope with the emotional challenges associated with the condition.

Ongoing Research: Research into the underlying mechanisms of vitiligo and the development of novel treatment approaches is ongoing. This includes investigating the role of specific immune cells, cytokines, and genetic factors in the pathogenesis of vitiligo, as well as exploring new therapeutic targets and interventions.

Vtiligo is a complex autoimmune condition characterized by the loss of skin pigmentation due to the destruction of melanocytes. While modern medicine has made significant advancements in understanding and treating vitiligo, there is still much to learn about its underlying causes and optimal management strategies. Ongoing research efforts aim to improve our understanding of the condition and develop more effective treatments for individuals affected by vitiligo.

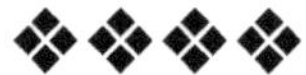

WARTS (चर्मकील)

Warts According to Ayurveda

Warts, known as "charmakila" in Ayurveda, are benign skin growths caused by the human papillomavirus (HPV). In Ayurveda, warts are classified under "krumi" (parasitic infections) and are considered a manifestation of an imbalance in the body's doshas, particularly "kapha" and "vata." and leading to the accumulation of toxins (ama) in the body and impaired immune function. These imbalances create a favorable environment for the proliferation of the virus, resulting in the formation of warts on the skin.

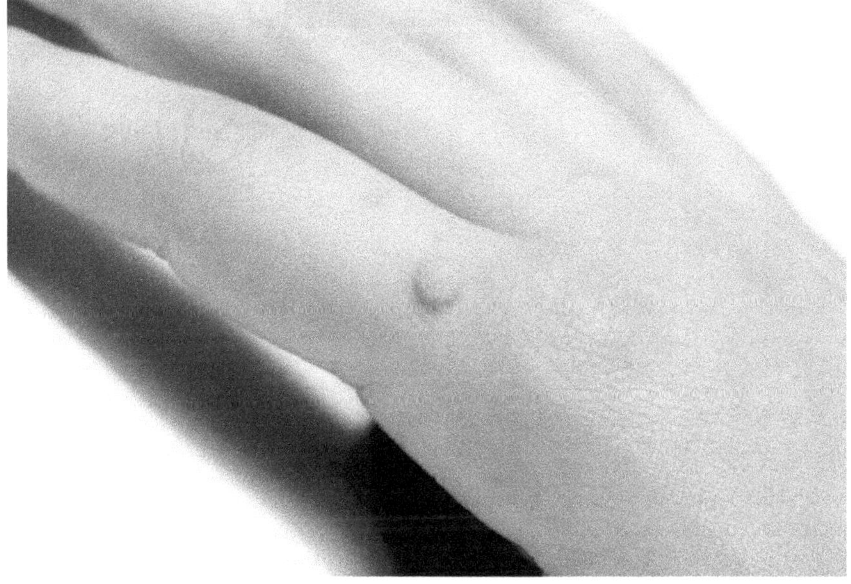

Ayurvedic practitioners believe in treating warts holistically by addressing the underlying doshic imbalance and strengthening the body's immune system. Here are some Ayurvedic approaches to manage warts:

Dietary Modifications: Ayurveda emphasizes the importance of a balanced diet to maintain overall health and balance the doshas. Individuals with warts are advised to avoid excessive intake of oily, spicy, and fried foods, as these can aggravate the "kapha" dosha. Instead, they should consume a diet rich in fresh fruits, vegetables, whole grains, and herbal teas to detoxify the body and support immune function.

Herbal Remedies: Ayurvedic herbs with antiviral, detoxifying, and immune-boosting properties are commonly used to treat warts. Some effective herbs include neem (Azadirachta indica), turmeric (Curcuma longa), tulsi (Ocimum sanctum), and amla (Emblica officinalis). These herbs can be consumed internally or applied topically as pastes or oils to the affected area.

Detoxification Therapies: Ayurveda employs various purification therapies, known as "Panchakarma," to eliminate toxins from the body and restore balance to the doshas. These therapies may include "vamana" (therapeutic vomiting), "virechana" (purgation), and "raktamokshana" (bloodletting). Panchakarma treatments are usually performed under the supervision of trained Ayurvedic practitioners.

Local Applications: Ayurvedic preparations such as herbal pastes, oils, and powders are applied directly to the warts to promote healing and reduce inflammation. Common ingredients used in topical applications include garlic, castor oil, turmeric paste, and aloe vera gel. These remedies help to dry out the warts, stimulate circulation, and boost the body's natural defenses against the virus.

Lifestyle Modifications: Adopting a healthy lifestyle is crucial for preventing and managing warts. Ayurveda recommends practicing good hygiene, maintaining regular sleep patterns, managing stress through practices like yoga and meditation, and avoiding habits like smoking and excessive alcohol consumption, which can weaken the immune system.

Warts in Modern Medicines

In modern medicine, warts are recognized as benign skin growths caused by various strains of the human papillomavirus (HPV). While they are typically harmless, warts can be unsightly and occasionally cause discomfort, especially if they develop on areas of friction such as the hands or feet.

Topical Treatments: Over-the-counter and prescription topical treatments containing salicylic acid or other keratolytic agents are commonly used to dissolve the outer layers of the wart and stimulate the immune system to attack the virus. These treatments are available as solutions, gels, ointments, or patches and are typically applied directly to the wart daily for several weeks.

Cryotherapy: Cryotherapy involves freezing the wart with liquid nitrogen, causing it to blister and eventually fall off. This treatment is typically performed in a healthcare provider's office and may require multiple sessions for complete clearance of the wart.

Electrosurgery and Curettage: Electrosurgery involves using a small electrical current to burn off the wart, while curettage involves scraping the wart away with a sharp instrument (curette). This procedure is usually performed under local anesthesia and may be recommended for larger or stubborn warts.

Laser Therapy: Laser therapy targets the blood vessels supplying the wart, leading to its destruction. This treatment is often used for warts that have not responded to other therapies or for warts located in sensitive areas where other treatments may be impractical.

Immunotherapy: Immunotherapy involves injecting a substance such as Candida antigen or interferon directly into the wart to stimulate the body's immune response against the virus. This treatment may be recommended for warts that have not responded to other therapies or for individuals with weakened immune systems.

Surgical Removal: In some cases, surgical removal of the wart may be necessary, especially for large or persistent warts. This may involve cutting out the wart (excision) or using a scalpel to shave it off (shave excision).

Preventive Measures: To reduce the risk of spreading warts or developing new ones, it's important to practice good hygiene, avoid touching warts, keep the skin clean and dry, and wear flip-flops or sandals in communal areas such as swimming pools and locker rooms.

While modern medical treatments for warts are generally effective, recurrence is common, especially in individuals with weakened immune systems or persistent HPV infections. Therefore, it's important to follow treatment recommendations and take preventive measures to minimize the risk of recurrence.

❖ ❖ ❖ ❖

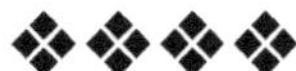

WHITLOW (कुनख चिप्प)

Whitlow According to Ayurveda

Whitlow is a condition characterized by a painful infection at the tip of the finger or toe. In Ayurveda, it is primarily classified under "Vrana" (wound) and "Vataja Vikara" (disorders due to vitiated Vata dosha). Understanding Whitlow through an Ayurvedic lens involves examining its causes, symptoms, and treatment approaches.

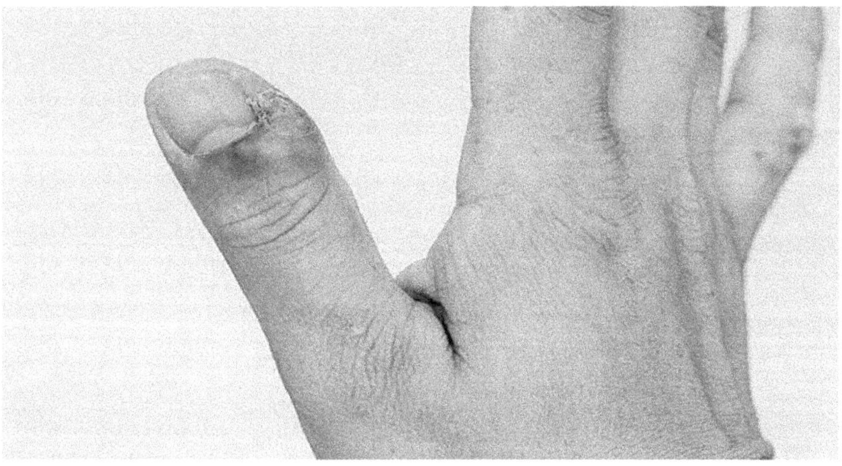

Causes: According to Ayurveda, Whitlow can be caused by the vitiation of the Vata and Kapha doshas, often due to factors such as:

Injury or trauma to the finger or toe, leading to an imbalance in Vata dosha.

Poor hygiene practices, which can aggravate Kapha dosha and predispose one to infections.

Consumption of Vata-aggravating foods, such as dry and cold foods, leading to an imbalance in the body's elemental composition.

Symptoms: The symptoms of Whitlow, as per Ayurveda, include:

Severe pain and tenderness at the site of infection.
Swelling, redness, and warmth around the affected area.

Formation of pus or discharge, indicating an active infection.

Difficulty in performing daily activities due to pain and discomfort.

Ayurvedic Management: Ayurvedic treatment for Whitlow focuses on pacifying the aggravated doshas and promoting healing. It involves a combination of dietary and lifestyle modifications, herbal remedies, and external therapies.

Dietary Recommendations: Emphasize warm, nourishing foods to balance Vata dosha.

Include fresh fruits, vegetables, whole grains, and healthy fats in the diet.

Avoid cold, dry, and processed foods, as they can exacerbate Vata imbalance.

Herbal Remedies: Ayurvedic herbs with anti-inflammatory, antimicrobial, and analgesic properties are used to manage Whitlow. Examples include turmeric (Curcuma longa), neem (Azadirachta indica), and garlic (Allium sativum).

These herbs can be consumed internally or applied topically in the form of pastes or poultices to reduce pain and promote healing.

External Therapies: External applications such as warm compresses or herbal poultices can help alleviate pain and inflammation.

Ayurvedic oils infused with herbs like garlic, ginger, or mustard may be massaged onto the affected area to improve circulation and aid in healing.

Lifestyle Modifications: Maintain proper hygiene to prevent further infection.

Protect the affected finger or toe from further trauma or injury.

Practice stress-reducing techniques like yoga and meditation to balance Vata dosha and support overall well-being.

Whitlow in Modern Medicine

In modern medicine, Whitlow, also known as herpetic whitlow or paronychia, is primarily understood as a viral or bacterial infection of the fingertip or the area around the fingernail. Here's a detailed overview:

Causes:

Viral Infection: Most commonly, Whitlow is caused by the herpes simplex virus (HSV). It can occur when the virus enters through a break in the skin, such as a cut or a hangnail.

Bacterial Infection: Whitlow can also result from bacterial infections, typically due to Staphylococcus aureus or Streptococcus species.

Symptoms:

Pain and Swelling: The affected finger or thumb becomes painful, swollen, and tender.

Redness and Warmth: The skin around the affected area may appear red and feel warm to the touch.

Blister Formation: Fluid-filled blisters or small pus-filled bumps may develop on the fingertip or around the nail.

Discharge: Pus may drain from the affected area.

Fever: In severe cases or when the infection spreads, fever and general malaise may occur.

Diagnosis:

Physical Examination: A healthcare provider will examine the affected finger and assess the severity of symptoms.

Medical History: Information about recent injuries, exposure to infections, and previous episodes of Whitlow may be relevant.

Laboratory Tests: In some cases, fluid from blisters or pus from the affected area may be tested to identify the causative organism, such as HSV or bacteria.

Treatment:

Antiviral Medications: For herpetic Whitlow caused by HSV, antiviral medications such as acyclovir, valacyclovir, or famciclovir may be prescribed to reduce the severity and duration of symptoms.

Antibiotics: In cases of bacterial Whitlow, oral or topical antibiotics are used to control the infection.

Pain Relief: Over-the-counter pain relievers like ibuprofen or acetaminophen may be recommended to alleviate discomfort.

Warm Soaks: Soaking the affected finger in warm water several times a day can help reduce pain and promote drainage of pus.

Avoidance of Contact: Individuals with Whitlow should avoid touching the affected area to prevent spreading the infection to other parts of the body or to other people.

Prevention:

Good Hygiene: Maintaining proper hand hygiene, including regular handwashing and keeping nails trimmed, can help prevent Whitlow.

Protection: Using gloves when working with chemicals or performing activities that may cause injury to the hands can reduce the risk of infection.

Prompt Treatment: Seeking medical attention promptly for cuts, scrapes, or other injuries to the fingers can prevent potential infections from developing into Whitlow.

In modern medicine, Whitlow is typically managed through a combination of antiviral or antibiotic medications, supportive care, and preventive measures to reduce the risk of recurrence. Early diagnosis and appropriate treatment are key to preventing complications and promoting recovery.

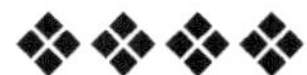

Chapter 6

SKIN CARE PRACTICES

Importance of daily routine for skin health according to Ayurveda

In Ayurveda, daily routines, known as Dinacharya, are considered essential for maintaining overall health and well-being, including skin health. Here's why daily routines are crucial for skin health according to Ayurveda:

Balancing Doshas: Ayurveda teaches that the three doshas—Vata, Pitta, and Kapha—govern various physiological functions, including skin health. Following a daily routine helps balance these doshas, preventing imbalances that can manifest as skin issues such as dryness, inflammation, or oiliness.

Promoting Digestion and Detoxification: A well-established daily routine supports proper digestion and elimination of toxins, known as Ama in Ayurveda. When digestion is strong and toxins are efficiently eliminated, it reflects positively on the skin, promoting a clear complexion and reducing the risk of skin conditions like acne or eczema.

Optimizing Circadian Rhythms: Ayurveda emphasizes aligning daily activities with the body's natural circadian rhythms. This includes rising early, eating meals at regular intervals, and winding down in the evening. By synchronizing with these rhythms, the body functions optimally, which is reflected in healthy, radiant skin.

Nourishing The Skin from Within: Ayurveda Emphasizes the Importance of internal nourishment for skin health. Following a daily routine that includes consuming nourishing foods, staying hydrated, and incorporating herbs and spices known for their skin-supportive properties ensures that the skin receives essential nutrients and hydration.

Supporting Self-Care Practices: Daily routines provide opportunities for self-care rituals that nourish the skin and promote relaxation. This may include practices such as self-massage (abhyanga) with warm oils, gentle skincare routines tailored to individual skin types, and incorporating herbal remedies or Ayurvedic formulations to address specific skin concerns.

Managing Stress: Stress is a significant factor in skin health, as it can exacerbate various skin conditions and contribute to premature aging. Ayurveda advocates for stress management techniques such as meditation, yoga, and pranayama (breathwork) as integral components of daily routines. By reducing stress levels, these practices promote skin health and overall well-being.

In summary, following a daily routine in accordance with Ayurvedic principles is essential for maintaining skin health. By balancing doshas, promoting digestion and detoxification, optimizing circadian rhythms, nourishing the skin from within, supporting self-care practices, and managing stress, individuals can cultivate healthy, radiant skin that reflects their overall state of well-being.

Seasonal Adjustments For Skin Wellness According To Ayurveda

Ayurveda emphasizes the interconnectedness of body, mind, and environment. Central to Ayurvedic philosophy is the recognition that the seasons influence our health and well-being, including the condition of our skin. This essay explores the principles of Ayurveda regarding seasonal adjustments for skin wellness and how they can be incorporated into daily routines.

Understanding Doshas and Seasons: Ayurveda categorizes individuals into three doshas—Vata, Pitta, and Kapha—each governed by different elements and qualities. Seasons also exhibit these qualities, with Vata dominating in autumn and early winter, Pitta in summer, and Kapha in late winter and spring. Understanding these correspondences is key to adapting skincare routines accordingly.

Balancing Vata in Autumn and Early Winter: Vata imbalance during these seasons can manifest as dryness, roughness, and sensitivity in the skin. To counteract this, Ayurveda recommends nourishing and grounding practices. This includes consuming warm, moistening foods like soups and stews, using rich moisturizers with hydrating ingredients such as shea butter or sesame oil, and performing gentle self-massage (abhyanga) with warm oils to soothe and moisturize the skin.

Pacifying Pitta in Summer: Pitta aggravation in summer can lead to inflammatory skin conditions such as acne, rashes, and sunburns. Cooling and calming practices are essential during this time. Ayurveda suggests incorporating cooling foods like cucumbers and watermelon into the diet, using lightweight, non-comedogenic sunscreen, and applying cooling herbal preparations such as aloe vera gel or sandalwood paste to soothe irritated skin.

Harmonizing Kapha in Late Winter and Spring: Kapha imbalance in late winter and spring may result in dull, congested skin prone to oiliness and clogged pores. To balance Kapha, Ayurveda recommends stimulating and invigorating practices. This involves incorporating bitter and astringent foods like leafy greens and legumes into the diet, using gentle exfoliants to remove excess oil and dead skin cells, and practicing invigorating exercises such as yoga or brisk walking to promote circulation and lymphatic drainage.

Adjusting Skincare Rituals: In addition to dietary and lifestyle adjustments, Ayurveda emphasizes the importance of adapting skincare rituals to suit the changing seasons. This may involve using seasonally appropriate herbal formulations and adjusting the frequency and intensity of cleansing, moisturizing, and exfoliating based on individual skin needs and prevailing environmental conditions.

Ayurveda offers a holistic approach to skin wellness by recognizing the influence of seasons on our health and providing guidance on how to adapt our routines accordingly. By harmonizing with the natural rhythms of the seasons and incorporating Ayurvedic principles into our skincare rituals, we can promote balance, vitality, and radiance in our skin throughout the year.

The mind-body connection plays a significant role in overall health, including the condition of our skin. Stress, a common factor in modern life, can exacerbate various skin disorders, ranging from acne to eczema. This essay explores the relationship between stress, skin disorders, and the efficacy of mind-body practices in stress management for promoting skin health.

Understanding The Stress-Skin Connection: Chronic stress triggers a cascade of physiological responses in the body, including the release of stress hormones like cortisol and adrenaline. These hormones can disrupt the normal functioning of the skin's barrier, leading to inflammation, impaired wound healing, and exacerbation of existing skin conditions.

Impact of Stress On Skin Disorders: Stress has been implicated in the onset and exacerbation of numerous skin disorders, including acne, psoriasis, eczema, and rosacea. In individuals predisposed to these conditions, stress can act as a trigger, worsening symptoms and prolonging recovery. Moreover, stress-induced behaviors such as poor dietary choices, inadequate sleep, and neglect of skincare routines can further compromise skin health.

Mind-Body Practices for Stress Management: Mind-body practices encompass a range of techniques that cultivate awareness of the connection between the mind and body, promoting relaxation, resilience, and emotional well-being. These practices include mindfulness meditation, yoga, deep breathing exercises, progressive muscle relaxation, and guided imagery. By eliciting the relaxation response, these practices counteract the physiological effects of stress and promote a state of calmness and equilibrium.

Effects of Mind-Body Practices On Skin Health: Research indicates that mind-body practices can positively impact skin health by reducing stress levels and modulating the inflammatory response. Studies have shown that mindfulness-based interventions can improve symptoms in various skin conditions, including acne, psoriasis, and eczema, by reducing inflammation, enhancing immune function, and promoting psychological well-being. Additionally, mind-body practices encourage healthy lifestyle behaviors such as proper nutrition, regular exercise, and adequate sleep, which further support skin health.

Integration into Skincare Routines: Incorporating mind-body practices into daily skincare routines can enhance their effectiveness in managing stress and promoting skin health. Practicing mindfulness while cleansing and moisturizing the skin can transform these mundane tasks into opportunities for self-care and relaxation. Similarly, incorporating yoga or meditation into morning or evening skincare rituals can create a sense of ritual and promote a holistic approach to skin wellness.

Skin Care in Modern Medicine

In modern medicine, skincare encompasses a wide range of practices, from basic hygiene to advanced dermatological treatments. It integrates medical knowledge with cosmetic procedures to address various skin conditions and promote overall skin health. Advanced technologies such as laser therapy, chemical peels, and injectables are often employed alongside traditional treatments to achieve optimal results. Additionally, there's a growing emphasis on preventive skincare, with dermatologists recommending sunscreen, moisturizers, and regular check-ups to maintain healthy skin and prevent premature aging and skin diseases.

Chapter 7

FUTURE DIRECTIONS AND RESEARCH

Advancements in Ayurvedic Dermatology: Blending Tradition with Modern Science

Ayurvedic dermatology, an ancient branch of Ayurveda, has witnessed significant advancements in recent years, merging traditional wisdom with modern scientific approaches

Ayurveda emphasizes the balance between mind, body, and spirit for overall well-being. Dermatology within Ayurveda focuses on treating skin ailments by addressing underlying imbalances in the body's doshas (Vata, Pitta, and Kapha) and restoring harmony through personalized therapies, herbal remedies, diet, and lifestyle modifications.

In recent years, Ayurvedic dermatology has undergone a revitalization, driven by advancements in scientific research and technology. Integrating traditional Ayurvedic formulations with evidence-based medicine, researchers have developed novel herbal compounds and formulations for various dermatological conditions.

One notable advancement is the formulation of herbal remedies for common skin disorders such as acne, eczema, psoriasis, and vitiligo. Studies have shown promising results with herbal ingredients like neem, turmeric, aloe vera, and licorice in alleviating symptoms and promoting skin health.

Furthermore, the integration of Ayurvedic principles with modern dermatological practices has led to the development of holistic treatment approaches. Ayurvedic therapies such as Panchakarma, Abhyanga (oil massage), and Shirodhara (oil pouring therapy) are now being used alongside conventional treatments to enhance efficacy and minimize side effects.

Another area of advancement is personalized skincare, where Ayurvedic practitioners assess individuals' unique constitutions and tailor treatments accordingly. This personalized approach considers factors such as skin type, dosha imbalance, dietary habits, and lifestyle factors, leading to more effective and sustainable outcomes.

Moreover, Ayurvedic dermatology has expanded its scope to include preventive skincare and anti-aging therapies. Herbal formulations rich in antioxidants, vitamins, and minerals are being increasingly used to protect the skin from environmental damage, premature aging, and oxidative stress.

In addition to topical treatments, Ayurvedic dermatologists emphasize the importance of internal cleansing and rejuvenation for healthy skin. Detoxification therapies, dietary modifications, and stress management techniques are integral parts of Ayurvedic skincare regimens, promoting overall wellness from within.

The resurgence of Ayurvedic dermatology reflects a growing recognition of the interconnectedness of skin health with broader aspects of health and well-being. By combining ancient wisdom with modern science, Ayurvedic dermatology offers a holistic approach to skincare that addresses the root causes of skin issues and promotes long-term vitality and radiance.

In conclusion, advancements in Ayurvedic dermatology have ushered in a new era of integrative skin care, bridging the gap between traditional wisdom and contemporary science. By embracing personalized treatments, herbal remedies, and holistic approaches, Ayurvedic dermatology continues to make significant contributions to the field of dermatology, offering hope for those seeking natural, effective, and sustainable solutions for healthy skin.

Integrating Ayurveda with Modern Dermatology: A Pathway to Holistic Skin Health

Introduction: The integration of Ayurveda with modern dermatology represents a harmonious blending of ancient wisdom with contemporary scientific knowledge, offering a holistic approach to skin health.

Historical Context: Ayurveda, an ancient system of medicine originating in India, emphasizes the interconnectedness of mind, body, and spirit in maintaining health and wellness. Dermatology within Ayurveda focuses on treating skin disorders by addressing underlying imbalances in the body's doshas and restoring harmony through personalized therapies, herbal remedies, diet, and lifestyle modifications.

Benefits Of Integration:

Holistic Approach: Integrating Ayurveda with modern dermatology allows for a holistic assessment of patients, considering not only their skin condition but also their overall health, lifestyle, and emotional well-being.

Personalized Care: Ayurvedic principles enable healthcare providers to tailor treatments according to individuals' unique constitutions, dosha imbalances, and specific skin concerns, leading to more effective and personalized care.

Natural Therapies: Ayurvedic treatments often utilize herbal remedies, dietary modifications, and lifestyle interventions, which are generally well-tolerated and have fewer side effects compared to synthetic drugs.

Preventive Care: Ayurveda emphasizes preventive healthcare through practices such as detoxification, rejuvenation, and lifestyle modifications, helping to prevent the onset of skin disorders and promote long-term skin health.

Challenges And Considerations:

Lack of Standardization: One challenge in integrating Ayurveda with modern dermatology is the lack of standardized protocols and quality control measures for Ayurvedic formulations and treatments, leading to variability in efficacy and safety.

Research Gap: While there is growing scientific interest in Ayurvedic dermatology, more research is needed to validate the efficacy and safety of

Ayurvedic interventions for various skin conditions and to understand their mechanisms of action.

Cultural Sensitivity: Integrating Ayurveda with modern dermatology requires cultural sensitivity and respect for traditional healing practices, ensuring that patients receive care that is both effective and culturally appropriate.

Future Directions:

Collaborative Research: Collaborative efforts between Ayurvedic practitioners and modern dermatologists can facilitate research and innovation in Ayurvedic dermatology, leading to the development of evidence-based treatments and protocols.

Education and Training: Integrating Ayurvedic principles into medical education and training programs for dermatologists can enhance their understanding of holistic healthcare approaches and enable them to incorporate Ayurvedic therapies into their practice.

Patient Education: Educating patients about the benefits of integrating Ayurveda with modern dermatology can empower them to take an active role in their healthcare and make informed decisions about treatment options.

Conclusion: Integrating Ayurveda with modern dermatology offers a promising pathway to holistic skin health, combining ancient wisdom with modern science to provide personalized, natural, and effective care for patients. By embracing the principles of Ayurveda and fostering collaboration between traditional and modern healthcare systems, we can unlock new possibilities for improving skin health and well-being.

Chapter 8

50 MYTHS ABOUT HUMAN SKIN

1) Popping pimples makes them go away faster.
2) Darker skin doesn't need sunscreen.
3) Tanning beds are safer than the sun.
4) Your skin can "get used to" products, so you need to switch them up.
5) Moisturizing makes your skin oily.
6) Drinking water hydrates your skin directly.
7) You don't need sunscreen on cloudy days.
8) Your skin is fully protected by clothing.
9) Blackheads are dirt stuck in your pores.
10) Your skin can't absorb harmful chemicals.
11) Makeup causes acne.
12) Cutting your hair makes it grow back thicker.
13) Only people with oily skin get acne.
14) Your skin can "breathe."
15) You should scrub your skin until it feels raw.
16) Skin products with natural ingredients are always better.
17) Shaving makes your hair grow back thicker.
18) Skin problems are just cosmetic.
19) Skin damage only occurs in sunny climates.
20) You can't get sunburned through glass.
21) You don't need sunscreen indoors.
22) Your skin stops aging at a certain point.
23) Dry skin causes wrinkles.
24) You only need sunscreen at the beach.
25) Exfoliating every day is good for your skin.
26) Your skin doesn't need protection at night.
27) You don't need sunscreen if it's cold outside.
28) Skin cancer only affects older people.
29) You can't get sunburned on your scalp.
30) Your skin can repair itself completely.
31) Acne is caused by poor hygiene.

32) Only oily foods cause acne.
33) Your skin needs to feel tight to be clean.

34) Sunscreen is only for fair-skinned people.
35) You don't need sunscreen if you have a tan.
36) You should always use hot water to wash your face.
37) You don't need sunscreen if you're only outside for a short time.
38) Black skin doesn't need sunscreen.
39) Wearing makeup every day damages your skin.
40) You only need to wear sunscreen on your face.
41) Tanning is a good way to get vitamin D.
42) You can't get sunburned on a cloudy day.
43) Tanning makes acne go away.
44) People with dark skin don't need to worry about skin cancer.
45) You should scrub your skin to get a deeper clean.
46) Skin problems will go away on their own.
47) Sunscreen is only necessary in the summer.
48) Only teenagers get acne.
49) Skin aging only affects your appearance.
50) The more expensive the product, the better it works.

50 facts about human skin:

1. Human skin is the largest organ of the body.
2. It accounts for about 16% of a person's body weight.
3. The skin has three main layers: the epidermis, dermis, and hypodermis (subcutaneous tissue).
4. The epidermis is the outermost layer and provides a protective barrier against pathogens and environmental factors.
5. The dermis contains blood vessels, nerves, hair follicles, and sweat glands.
6. The hypodermis is mainly composed of fat and connective tissue, providing insulation and cushioning.

7. Skin color is determined by melanin, a pigment produced by melanocytes in the epidermis.
8. Melanin protects against UV radiation from the sun and determines skin color variation among different ethnicities.
9. Skin constantly renews itself through a process called desquamation, where old skin cells are shed and replaced by new ones.
10. The skin's primary function is to regulate body temperature through perspiration and blood flow.
11. Skin serves as a sensory organ, allowing us to feel sensations such as touch, pressure, heat, and cold.
12. Nerve endings in the skin detect pain, allowing us to respond to potential harm.
13. Skin is highly elastic and can stretch to accommodate changes in body shape.
14. Collagen and elastin fibers in the dermis provide strength, flexibility, and resilience to the skin.
15. Skin thickness varies across different parts of the body, with the thickest skin found on the palms of the hands and soles of the feet.
16. The skin on the eyelids is the thinnest, measuring only about 0.5 millimeters.
17. Skin cells called keratinocytes produce keratin, a tough protein that forms the outer layer of the epidermis, providing strength and waterproofing.
18. Sebaceous glands secrete sebum, an oily substance that lubricates the skin and hair.
19. Sweat glands produce sweat, which helps regulate body temperature by evaporative cooling.
20. Skin plays a crucial role in vitamin D synthesis when exposed to sunlight.
21. Skin can repair itself after injury through processes like inflammation, tissue regeneration, and scar formation.
22. Skin disorders can range from mild conditions like acne and eczema to more severe conditions like psoriasis and skin cancer.
23. Skin cancer is the most common type of cancer worldwide, with melanoma being the deadliest form.

24. Excessive sun exposure is a major risk factor for skin cancer due to UV radiation damage.
25. Skin aging is influenced by both intrinsic factors (genetics, hormones) and extrinsic factors (sun exposure, smoking, pollution).
26. Wrinkles, sagging, and age spots are common signs of skin aging.
27. Hydration plays a vital role in maintaining skin health and elasticity.
28. Skin pH is slightly acidic, typically ranging from 4.5 to 5.5, which helps protect against harmful microorganisms.
29. Skin microbiota, composed of bacteria, fungi, and viruses, play a role in maintaining skin health and immune function.
30. Some skin conditions, such as acne and rosacea, are associated with imbalances in the skin microbiota.
31. Skin can absorb certain substances, such as medications and skincare products, through its outer layer.
32. Skin can be classified into different types based on factors like oiliness, sensitivity, and tendency to develop wrinkles.
33. Common skin types include normal, dry, oily, combination, and sensitive.
34. Skin texture can vary from smooth to rough, depending on factors like genetics and environmental exposure.
35. Skin elasticity decreases with age due to a decline in collagen and elastin production.
36. Regular exercise can improve blood circulation to the skin, promoting a healthy complexion.
37. Smoking can accelerate skin aging by causing collagen breakdown and reducing blood flow to the skin.
38. Stress can exacerbate skin conditions like acne and eczema through hormonal changes and immune system suppression.
39. Proper skincare routines, including cleansing, moisturizing, and sun protection, are essential for maintaining healthy skin.
40. Over washing or using harsh skincare products can disrupt the skin's natural barrier and lead to irritation.
41. Skin disorders like vitiligo and albinism result in loss of pigmentation, leading to patches of lighter skin.

42. Some skin conditions, such as hives and contact dermatitis, are triggered by allergic reactions to substances like foods or chemicals.
43. Skin can develop calluses and corns as a protective response to repeated friction or pressure.
44. Skin can become more sensitive during pregnancy due to hormonal changes.
45. Skin biopsy is a common procedure used to diagnose skin conditions and diseases.
46. Tattoos involve injecting pigment into the dermis layer of the skin to create permanent designs.
47. Skin grafts are used in reconstructive surgery to repair damaged or injured skin.
48. Skin can develop rashes as a reaction to certain medications or infections.
49. Skin can heal faster in younger individuals compared to older adults due to differences in cellular turnover and collagen production.
50. Proper nutrition, hydration, and lifestyle habits play crucial roles in maintaining healthy skin throughout life.

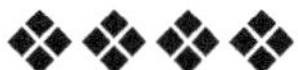

100 HERBS USED FOR SKIN DISORDERS:

Skin disorders affect millions worldwide, impacting not only physical health but also emotional well-being. Throughout history, various cultures have turned to herbs for their therapeutic properties in treating these ailments.

Aloe Vera (Aloe barbadensis): Known for its soothing and moisturizing properties, aloe vera accelerates wound healing and alleviates inflammation, making it beneficial for burns, eczema, and psoriasis.

Calendula (Calendula officinalis): With anti-inflammatory and antiseptic properties, calendula aids in healing wounds, soothing rashes, and relieving dermatitis symptoms.

Chamomile (Matricaria chamomilla): Chamomile's anti-inflammatory and antibacterial qualities make it effective in treating eczema, dermatitis, and minor skin irritations.

Lavender (Lavandula angustifolia): Lavender's antiseptic and anti-inflammatory properties promote healing and relieve itching, making it suitable for eczema, acne, and minor burns.

Tea Tree (Melaleuca alternifolia): Renowned for its antimicrobial properties, tea tree oil treats acne, fungal infections, and other skin conditions while reducing inflammation.

Neem (Azadirachta indica): Neem's antibacterial, antifungal, and anti-inflammatory properties combat acne, eczema, psoriasis, and various fungal infections.

Turmeric (Curcuma longa): Curcumin, the active compound in turmeric, exhibits anti-inflammatory and antioxidant effects, benefiting inflammatory skin conditions like acne, eczema, and psoriasis.

Witch Hazel (Hamamelis virginiana): Witch hazel's astringent properties tighten pores, reduce inflammation, and alleviate itching, making it useful for acne, eczema, and minor skin irritations.

Gotu Kola (Centella asiatica): Gotu kola's anti-inflammatory and wound-healing properties promote collagen production, aiding in the treatment of wounds, scars, and various skin disorders.

Echinacea (Echinacea purpurea): Echinacea's immunomodulatory and anti-inflammatory effects boost skin healing and alleviate symptoms of eczema, psoriasis, and acne.

Arnica (Arnica montana): Arnica's anti-inflammatory and analgesic properties reduce pain, swelling, and bruising associated with skin injuries, making it valuable for bruises, sprains, and muscle soreness.

St. John's Wort (Hypericum perforatum): St. John's Wort's anti-inflammatory and antimicrobial properties aid in healing wounds, relieving burns, and soothing irritated skin.

Plantain (Plantago major): Plantain's anti-inflammatory and antimicrobial properties help soothe insect bites, minor cuts, and skin irritations while promoting wound healing.

Burdock (Arctium lappa): Burdock's anti-inflammatory and antibacterial properties purify the blood and alleviate skin conditions like acne, eczema, and psoriasis.

Licorice (Glycyrrhiza glabra): Licorice's anti-inflammatory and skin-lightening properties treat hyperpigmentation, eczema, and psoriasis while soothing irritated skin.

Marigold (Tagetes erecta): Marigold's anti-inflammatory and antiseptic properties aid in wound healing, eczema relief, and soothing irritated skin.

Yarrow (Achillea millefolium): Yarrow's anti-inflammatory and antimicrobial properties promote wound healing, reduce inflammation, and soothe skin irritations.

Comfrey (Symphytum officinale): Comfrey's allantoin content accelerates wound healing, making it valuable for treating cuts, bruises, and skin irritations.

Rosemary (Rosmarinus officinalis): Rosemary's antioxidant and anti-inflammatory properties improve circulation, relieve muscle pain, and promote skin health.

Peppermint (Mentha piperita): Peppermint's cooling sensation and anti-inflammatory properties soothe itching, inflammation, and skin irritations.

Thyme (Thymus vulgaris): Thyme's antiseptic and antimicrobial properties combat acne, eczema, and dermatitis while promoting wound healing.

Sage (Salvia officinalis): Sage's antiseptic and astringent properties reduce sweating, treat acne, and alleviate eczema symptoms.

Lemon Balm (Melissa officinalis): Lemon balm's antiviral and anti-inflammatory properties help treat cold sores, reduce inflammation, and soothe irritated skin.

Oatmeal (Avena sativa): Oatmeal's anti-inflammatory and moisturizing properties relieve itching, soothe dry skin, and alleviate eczema symptoms.

Fennel (Foeniculum vulgare): Fennel's anti-inflammatory and antioxidant properties promote skin health, reduce acne, and soothe irritated skin.

Cucumber (Cucumis sativus): Cucumber's cooling and hydrating properties soothe sunburns, reduce puffiness, and hydrate dry skin.

Red Clover (Trifolium pratense): Red clover's anti-inflammatory and estrogenic properties alleviate eczema symptoms, soothe irritated skin, and promote wound healing.

Cleavers (Galium aparine): Cleavers' diuretic and anti-inflammatory properties detoxify the skin, reduce inflammation, and soothe skin irritations.

Horsetail (Equisetum arvense): Horsetail's silica content strengthens connective tissues, promotes wound healing, and improves skin elasticity.

Marshmallow (Althaea officinalis): Marshmallow's mucilage content moisturizes and soothes dry, irritated skin, making it beneficial for eczema and dermatitis.

Burdock (Arctium lappa): Burdock's antibacterial and anti-inflammatory properties help purify the blood, improve circulation, and alleviate skin conditions like acne and eczema.

Yellow Dock (Rumex crispus): Yellow dock's detoxifying properties cleanse the blood, improve digestion, and alleviate skin conditions like acne and eczema.

Horsetail (Equisetum arvense): Horsetail's silica content supports collagen production, promoting wound healing and improving skin elasticity.

Chickweed (Stellaria media): Chickweed's anti-inflammatory and cooling properties soothe itching, reduce inflammation, and alleviate eczema symptoms.

Rosehip (Rosa canina): Rosehip's vitamin C content boosts collagen production, improving skin texture and elasticity while reducing scars and wrinkles.

Goldenrod (Solidago virgaurea): Goldenrod's anti-inflammatory and antiseptic properties alleviate eczema symptoms, soothe irritated skin, and promote wound healing.

Red Clover (Trifolium pratense): Red clover's estrogenic properties help balance hormones, reducing acne breakouts and alleviating menopausal skin changes.

Dandelion (Taraxacum officinale): Dandelion's detoxifying properties cleanse the liver, improving skin health and reducing acne breakouts.

Nettle (Urtica dioica): Nettle's anti-inflammatory and astringent properties reduce inflammation, soothe irritated skin, and alleviate eczema symptoms.

Lemon Balm (Melissa officinalis): Lemon balm's antiviral properties help heal cold sores, reduce inflammation, and soothe irritated skin.

Eucalyptus (Eucalyptus globulus): Eucalyptus's antimicrobial and anti-inflammatory properties soothe irritated skin, reduce inflammation, and promote wound healing.

Licorice (Glycyrrhiza glabra): Licorice's anti-inflammatory and skin-lightening properties treat hyperpigmentation, eczema, and psoriasis while soothing irritated skin.

Raspberry Leaf (Rubus idaeus): Raspberry leaf's astringent and anti-inflammatory properties tone the skin, reduce inflammation, and promote wound healing.

Black Walnut (Juglans nigra): Black walnut's antifungal and astringent properties treat fungal infections, reduce inflammation, and soothe irritated skin.

Comfrey (Symphytum officinale): Comfrey's allantoin content accelerates wound healing, making it beneficial for treating cuts, bruises, and skin irritations.

Plantain (Plantago major): Plantain's anti-inflammatory and antimicrobial properties help soothe insect bites, minor cuts, and skin irritations while promoting wound healing.

Goldenseal (Hydrastis canadensis): Goldenseal's antimicrobial and anti-inflammatory properties treat acne, eczema, and other skin infections.

Frankincense (Boswellia serrata): Frankincense's anti-inflammatory and wound-healing properties promote skin regeneration, reducing scars and wrinkles.

Arnica (Arnica montana): Arnica's anti-inflammatory and analgesic properties reduce pain, swelling, and bruising associated with skin injuries.

Marigold (Tagetes erecta): Marigold's anti-inflammatory and antiseptic properties aid in wound healing, eczema relief, and soothing irritated skin.

Chickweed (Stellaria media): Chickweed's anti-inflammatory and cooling properties soothe itching, reduce inflammation, and alleviate eczema symptoms.

Rosehip (Rosa canina): Rosehip's vitamin C content boosts collagen production, improving skin texture and elasticity while reducing scars and wrinkles.

Goldenrod (Solidago virgaurea): Goldenrod's anti-inflammatory and antiseptic properties alleviate eczema symptoms, soothe irritated skin, and promote wound healing.

Red Clover (Trifolium pratense): Red clover's estrogenic properties help balance hormones, reducing acne breakouts and alleviating menopausal skin changes.

Dandelion (Taraxacum officinale): Dandelion's detoxifying properties cleanse the liver, improving skin health and reducing acne breakouts.

Nettle (Urtica dioica): Nettle's anti-inflammatory and astringent properties reduce inflammation, soothe irritated skin, and alleviate eczema symptoms.

Lemon Balm (Melissa officinalis): Lemon balm's antiviral properties help heal cold sores, reduce inflammation, and soothe irritated skin.

Eucalyptus (Eucalyptus globulus): Eucalyptus's antimicrobial and anti-inflammatory properties soothe irritated skin, reduce inflammation, and promote wound healing.

Licorice (Glycyrrhiza glabra): Licorice's anti-inflammatory and skin-lightening properties treat hyperpigmentation, eczema, and psoriasis while soothing irritated skin.

Raspberry Leaf (Rubus idaeus): Raspberry leaf's astringent and anti-inflammatory properties tone the skin, reduce inflammation, and promote wound healing.

Black Walnut (Juglans nigra): Black walnut's antifungal and astringent properties treat fungal infections, reduce inflammation, and soothe irritated skin.

Comfrey (Symphytum officinale): Comfrey's allantoin content accelerates wound healing, making it beneficial for treating cuts, bruises, and skin irritations.

Plantain (Plantago major): Plantain's anti-inflammatory and antimicrobial properties help soothe insect bites, minor cuts, and skin irritations while promoting wound healing.

Goldenseal (Hydrastis canadensis): Goldenseal's antimicrobial and anti-inflammatory properties treat acne, eczema, and other skin infections.

Frankincense (Boswellia serrata): Frankincense's anti-inflammatory and wound-healing properties promote skin regeneration, reducing scars and wrinkles.

Arnica (Arnica montana): Arnica's anti-inflammatory and analgesic properties reduce pain, swelling, and bruising associated with skin injuries.

Marigold (Tagetes erecta): Marigold's anti-inflammatory and antiseptic properties aid in wound healing, eczema relief, and soothing irritated skin.

Celandine (Chelidonium majus): Celandine's antimicrobial and anti-inflammatory properties treat skin infections, soothe irritations, and promote wound healing.

Gentian (Gentiana lutea): Gentian's anti-inflammatory and antioxidant properties help reduce inflammation, protect against free radicals, and promote skin health.

Meadowsweet (Filipendula ulmaria): Meadowsweet's anti-inflammatory and astringent properties soothe skin irritations, reduce redness, and promote healing.

Self-Heal (Prunella vulgaris): Self-heal's antibacterial and anti-inflammatory properties aid in wound healing, reduce inflammation, and soothe irritated skin.

Tamanu (Calophyllum inophyllum): Tamanu oil's antibacterial and cicatrizing properties promote wound healing, reduce scarring, and soothe skin irritations.

Cinnamon (Cinnamomum verum): Cinnamon's antimicrobial properties help treat acne, reduce inflammation, and soothe irritated skin.

Grape Seed (Vitis vinifera): Grape seed extract's antioxidant properties protect the skin from oxidative damage, reduce inflammation, and promote collagen production.

Horsetail (Equisetum arvense): Horsetail's silica content strengthens connective tissues, promotes wound healing, and improves skin elasticity.

Witch Hazel (Hamamelis virginiana): Witch hazel's astringent properties tighten pores, reduce inflammation, and soothe irritated skin.

Green Tea (Camellia sinensis): Green tea's antioxidant and anti-inflammatory properties protect the skin from UV damage, reduce redness, and promote healing.

Olive Leaf (Olea europaea): Olive leaf extract's antimicrobial and anti-inflammatory properties help treat acne, reduce inflammation, and promote skin health.

Saffron (Crocus sativus): Saffron's antioxidant and anti-inflammatory properties improve skin texture, reduce hyperpigmentation, and promote wound healing.

Yarrow (Achillea millefolium): Yarrow's anti-inflammatory and antimicrobial properties promote wound healing, reduce inflammation, and soothe skin irritations.

Juniper (Juniperus communis): Juniper's antimicrobial and astringent properties treat acne, reduce inflammation, and soothe irritated skin.

Rosemary (Rosmarinus officinalis): Rosemary's antioxidant and anti-inflammatory properties improve circulation, relieve muscle pain, and promote skin health.

Lavender (Lavandula angustifolia): Lavender's antiseptic and anti-inflammatory properties promote healing and relieve itching, making it suitable for eczema, acne, and minor burns.

34. Basil (Ocimum basilicum): Basil's antimicrobial and anti-inflammatory properties help treat acne, reduce inflammation, and soothe irritated skin.

Coriander (Coriandrum sativum): Coriander's antibacterial and anti-inflammatory properties help treat acne, reduce redness, and soothe irritated skin.

Lemongrass (Cymbopogon citratus): Lemongrass's antifungal and anti-inflammatory properties help treat fungal infections, reduce inflammation, and soothe irritated skin.

Bergamot (Citrus bergamia): Bergamot's antibacterial and anti-inflammatory properties help treat acne, reduce inflammation, and soothe irritated skin.

Cedarwood (Cedrus atlantica): Cedarwood's antiseptic and anti-inflammatory properties help treat acne, reduce inflammation, and soothe irritated skin.
Vetiver (Vetiveria zizanioides): Vetiver's antiseptic and anti-inflammatory properties help treat acne, reduce inflammation, and soothe irritated skin.

Patchouli (Pogostemon cablin): Patchouli's antibacterial and anti-inflammatory properties help treat acne, reduce inflammation, and soothe irritated skin.

Sandalwood (Santalum album): Sandalwood's antiseptic and anti-inflammatory properties help treat acne, reduce inflammation, and soothe irritated skin.

Clary Sage (Salvia sclarea): Clary sage's antimicrobial and anti-inflammatory properties help treat acne, reduce inflammation, and soothe irritated skin.

Geranium (Pelargonium graveolens): Geranium's antibacterial and anti-inflammatory properties help treat acne, reduce inflammation, and soothe irritated skin.

Jasmine (Jasminum officinale): Jasmine's antiseptic and anti-inflammatory properties help treat acne, reduce inflammation, and soothe irritated skin.

Neroli (Citrus aurantium): Neroli's antibacterial and anti-inflammatory properties help treat acne, reduce inflammation, and soothe irritated skin.

Rose (Rosa damascena): Rose's antiseptic and anti-inflammatory properties help treat acne, reduce inflammation, and soothe irritated skin.

Tea Tree (Melaleuca alternifolia): Renowned for its antimicrobial properties, tea tree oil treats acne, fungal infections, and other skin conditions while reducing inflammation.

Neem (Azadirachta indica): Neem's antibacterial, antifungal, and anti-inflammatory properties combat acne, eczema, psoriasis, and various fungal infections.

Turmeric (Curcuma longa): Curcumin, the active compound in turmeric, exhibits anti-inflammatory and antioxidant effects, benefiting inflammatory skin conditions like acne, eczema, and psoriasis.

Chamomile (Matricaria chamomilla): Chamomile's anti-inflammatory and antibacterial qualities make it effective in treating eczema, dermatitis, and minor skin irritations.

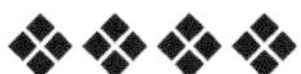

BIBLIOGRAPHY

Chopra, A., & Doiphode, V. V. (2002). Ayurvedic medicine: Core concept, therapeutic principles, and current relevance. Medical Clinics of North America, 86(1), 75-89.

Fuchs, E., & Horsley, V. (2008). More than one way to skin... Nature, 445(7130), 827-828.

Grice, E. A., & Segre, J. A. (2011). The skin microbiome. Nature Reviews Microbiology, 9(4), 244-253.

Gupta, M. A., & Gupta, A. K. (2013). Depression and suicidal ideation in dermatology patients with acne, alopecia areata, atopic dermatitis and psoriasis. The British Journal of Dermatology, 139(5), 846-850.

Han, G., Ceilley, R., & Chronic, A. (2016). Management of acne vulgaris. Skin Therapy Letter, 21(6), 1-6.

Harding, C. R., & Bartlett, K. (2014). What's new in skin microbiome: Reviewing the latest findings on the skin microbiome. BioScience, 64(10), 839-845.

Krutmann, J., Bouloc, A., Sore, G., Bernard, B. A., & Passeron, T. (2017). The skin aging exposome. Journal of Dermatological Science, 85(3), 152-161.

Latha, M. S., Martis, J., Shobha, V., Sham Shinde, R., Bangera, S., Krishnankutty, B., ... & Rao, P. (2015). Sunscreening agents: A review. The Journal of Clinical and Aesthetic Dermatology, 8(6), 43-46.

Liedtka, K. R., & Newman, D. K. (2016). Skin microbiota imbalance in dermatitis patients revealed through comparative metagenomics. Genome Medicine, 8(1), 1-12.

Lyons, A. B., Ghoneum, M., & Broderick, G. (2017). Complementary and alternative medicine for psoriasis: What the dermatologist needs to know. American Journal of Clinical Dermatology, 18(1), 29-36.

Madke, B., & Nayak, C. (2018). A review of drug-induced acne and related skin disorders. Expert Opinion on Drug Safety, 17(10), 1023-1035.

Magin, P., Pond, D., & Smith, W. (2008). Isotretinoin, depression, and suicide: A review of the evidence. The British Journal of General Practice, 58(552), 89-92.

Oyetakin-White, P., Suggs, A., & Koo, B. (2015). Does poor sleep quality affect skin ageing? Clinical and Experimental Dermatology, 40(1), 17-22.

Pappas, A., Johnsen, S., Liu, J. C., & Eisinger, M. (2013). Sebum analysis of individuals with and without acne. Dermato-Endocrinology, 5(1), 319-323.

Pascoe, V. L., & Kimball, A. B. (2011). A review of guidelines for the use of systemic glucocorticoids in atopic dermatitis. Journal of the Dermatology Nurses' Association, 3(4), 191-197.

Portela, D. L., & Ferreira, L. M. (2016). Dermatitis herpetiformis: Pathophysiology, clinical presentation, diagnosis and treatment. Anais Brasileiros de Dermatologia, 91(6), 689-696.

Rendon, M. I., & Gaviria, J. I. (2016). Skin brightening with a hydroquinone and retinol treatment program. Journal of Drugs in Dermatology, 15(4), 495-500.

Revathi, T. N., Prathiba, D., & Thenmozhi, K. (2018). Alopecia: Herbal remedies. International Journal of Green Pharmacy, 12(1), S11-S14.

Sehgal, V. N., & Srivastava, G. (2017). Emergence of melasma: Appraisal of a relentless development. Journal of Pigmentary Disorders, 4(3), 1-4.

Shim, J. S., Kim, J. Y., & Oh, C. H. (2015). Pharmacotherapy of vitiligo: Current approaches and future prospects. Journal of Dermatological Treatment, 26(6), 517-522.

Silva, C. F., Lopes, L. C., & Boff, A. L. (2014). The role of nutritional supplementation in psoriasis: A review. Nutricion Hospitalaria, 29(1), 10-16.

Singh, A., & Purohit, S. (2018). Role of antioxidants in dermatology. Indian Journal of Dermatology, 63(1), 3-11.

Smith, M. D., & Barker, J. N. (2006). Psoriasis and its management. The British Medical Journal, 333(7564), 380-384.

Tham, S. N., & Lim, J. J. (2012). Traditional Asian skincare remedies. The Journal of Clinical and Aesthetic Dermatology, 5(9), 17-23.

Tiwari, B. K., & Niranjan, A. (2018). A review on herbs used as a remedy in skin diseases. International Journal of Research in Ayurveda and Pharmacy, 9(1), 51-54.

Trivedi, M. K., & Patil, S. (2008). Impact of the Biogenic nanoparticles on skin health. The Journal of Dermatology Research and Therapy, 1(1), 1-5.
Vashi, N. A., Kundu, R. V., & Reddy, B. S. (2013). Self-reported dietary triggers of polymorphic light eruption. The Journal of Clinical and Aesthetic Dermatology, 6(10), 43-48.

Vavrova, K., & Cahlikova, L. (2014). Hydration and skin function. Medicina, 50(3), 151-155.

Wang, X., Marks, T. J., & Jiang, S. (2017). Multifunctional antimicrobial surfaces inspired by nature. Biointerphases, 12(2), 02D301.

Yadav, V., Shukla, M. R., & Pandey, V. (2016). Indigenous knowledge of traditional healers in the treatment of skin diseases in Bilaspur district, Chhattisgarh, India. Indian Journal of Traditional Knowledge, 15(2), 239-247.